WORKBOOK
for

ACHIEVING TRUE WELLNESS IN A WORLD OF HEALTH LIES

Unveiling the Confusion, Myths, and Deceptions Keeping You from Lasting Health

Second Edition

by

DR. JACKIE MCKOOL

Copyright ©2025 by Dr. Jackie McKool. Achieving True Wellness in a World Of Health Lies: Unveiling the Confusion, Myths, and Deceptions Keeping You from Lasting Health, Second Edition

Published by Leadership Books, Inc. Las Vegas, NV – New York, NY

LeadershipBooks.com

ISBN
Hardback: 978-1-965401-72-9
Paperback: 978-1-965401-73-6
eBook: 978-1-965401-74-3
Workbook: 978-1-951648-92-3

All Rights Reserved. No part of this publication may be reproduced, distributed, or transmitted in any form or by any means, including photocopying, recording, or other electronic or mechanical methods without the prior written permission of the publisher, except in the case of brief quotations embodied in critical reviews and certain other noncommercial uses permitted by copyright law.

Leadership Books, Inc. is committed to publishing works of quality and integrity. In that spirit, we are proud to offer this book to our readers; however, the story, the experiences, and the words are the authors alone. The conversations in the book all come from the author's recollections, not word-for-word transcripts. All of the events are true to the best of the author's memory. The author, in no way, represents any company, corporation, or brand mentioned herein. The views expressed are solely those of the author.

The information presented is the author's opinion and does not constitute any health or medical advice. The content of this workbook is for informational purposes only and is not intended to diagnose, treat, cure, or prevent any condition or disease.

A Note from the Author

Thank you for picking up this second edition. While the heart and message of this book remain the same, you'll notice a few updates designed to improve your reading experience. The chapters have been thoughtfully reordered for better flow and clarity, and the book has been given a new title and cover design to more accurately reflect its message and purpose.

These changes were made in response to valuable reader feedback and my own continued growth and insight since the original release. I pray this edition serves you even more deeply on your journey toward true wellness and wholeness.

In grace and truth, Dr. Jackie McKool

*I dedicate this workbook
to my dad,
Robert McKool,*

in whose footsteps I have followed as a teacher. Thank you, Pops, for instilling in me a desire to share with others what we are most passionate about—

for you, it was flying; for me, it's health and wellness.

WORKBOOK
for

ACHIEVING TRUE WELLNESS IN A WORLD OF HEALTH LIES

Unveiling the Confusion, Myths, and Deceptions Keeping You from Lasting Health

Second Edition

TABLE OF CONTENTS

INTRODUCTION: Understanding Your Study Guide......................................ix

PART ONE: CLEARING THE MUDDIED WATERS: A PARADIGM SHIFT TOWARD TRUE WELLNESS..........5

Chapter 1: The Truth About Where Health Comes From 7

Chapter 2: A Paradigm Shift—What Wellness Is NOT 13

Chapter 3: The Paradigm Shift Continued—What Wellness IS 19

Chapter 4: Caring for Your Spiritual, Mental, and Emotional Health..............27

Chapter 5: Physical Health 41

Chapter 6: Inflammatory versus Non-Inflammatory Foods.................55

PART TWO: A LITTLE ANATOMY CAN GO A LONG WAY.............. 63

Chapter 7: Four Organs and Systems of the Body That Can Extend Your Health!......................................65

Chapter 8: The Connection Between Trauma & Addiction "Which Came First, The Chicken or The Egg?"(Stress or Addiction?).........73

PART THREE: TRUTH VS. DECEPTION: LIVE A LIFE OF HEALTH AND EMPOWERMENT!.......................79

Chapter 9: The Truths—Open Your Eyes and Ears!..............................81

PART FOUR: OUTSIDE HELP: THOSE WHO CAN WALK ALONGSIDE YOU AND THE TOOLS AVAILABLE TO YOU 89

Chapter 10: The Truth About Natural Healthcare Practitioners, Building Your Healthcare Team 91

Chapter 11: The Truth about Supplements 97

Chapter 12: The Truth about Wholistic Health Tests 103

Conclusion 109

Appendix-A: Suggested Reading And Resources 111

Appendix-B: Wholistic Goals 115

Appendix-C: Food Log 117

About Dr. Jackie Mckool 125

Understanding Your Study Guide

Additional features for each session include:

REVIEW Each session begins with a quick recap of the previous session and how its teachings have begun to impact our lives.

KEY VERSE Each session has a key bible verse to memorize. Do it out loud and have fun!

VIDEO-STREAMING Each session has a video-streaming lesson to present specifically designed material. Enjoy!

INTRODUCTION Each session has an introductory, read-aloud paragraph(s) to kick off and focus the group's discussion.

QUESTIONS FOR DISCUSSION Each session has multiple questions corresponding chapter-by-chapter to the book, *Achieving True Wellness in a World of Health Lies*. These questions are designed to encourage open and honest discussion to elicit a more comprehensive understanding of the wholistic and biblical concepts, texts, and lessons taught and illustrated in the book; and to create a comfortable learning experience.

GUIDE FOR LEADERS

Open each session in prayer. Pray that you hear God's voice guiding you through each lesson. Ask Him to push aside your own desires of what to say and allow you to speak only what He would have you say for each lesson. Pray for the current week's specific lesson/topic. Ask Him to give the participants ears to hear, eyes to see, and a heart to obey His truths about their wholistic health—mental, emotional, physical, and spiritual.

Take time during each lesson to have the participants write down why they decided to pursue this study, if they have not already done so, reflecting on what they hope to get out of each lesson and what changes they are prepared to commit to making. Ask if anyone is willing to share their answers.

Take time to discuss, as a group, the answers to the questions for each lesson.

Instruct the group to watch the video, read the next chapter, and answer all of the questions for next week.

Ask for prayer requests—ideally pertaining to them and their health journey.

Close in prayer.

INTRODUCTION

VIDEO STREAMING: INTRODUCTION

This workbook is designed to accompany *Achieving True Wellness in a World of Health Lies: Unveiling the Confusion, Myths, and Deceptions Keeping You from Lasting Health*. The book of Proverbs says, "A hard worker has plenty of food, but a person who chases fantasies has no sense." (Proverbs 12:11 NLT)

Reading the book is enlightening, but if at least some of the principles are not applied, I have failed you. The book's objective is to first educate you on the real truths about health and wellness. But it shouldn't stop there. Second, I hope it encourages you, if not flat out excites you, to know that your health really is in your control! But most of all, I pray that it empowers you to walk out into all that God has called you to be and do, with freedom! This workbook is a tool to help you accomplish that.

Take your time with it. Health and healing are a process—in fact, they are a lifetime process. There are new things to be discovered about your health all the time. After all, we are not stagnant beings. Each day, our bodies change just a little bit more, for better or worse, fast or slow. What you did 10 years ago or even last month to take care of your temple—the only body God gave you to steward—is going to be different from what you do today, or next year, or 10 years from now.

My prayer is that this workbook will help you take what you just read and watched, which might have felt like drinking from a water hose—I know, I've been there—and apply it. To help break all this information down into bite-sized pieces.

Once you have watched the videos, read through the book, and worked through this workbook, write down your game plan, commit to it, and then tuck it away for a season. Revisit it every so often—whether it be once a quarter, once a year, or once every 5 years. Or maybe when you feel you have become stagnant and need a boost, revisit this information to remind yourself why you were doing what you were doing. The book, workbook, and videos do not have to be a one-and-done. They can be utilized over and over again for a refresher when needed. Your health goals will change over time, so I encourage you to revisit all of this.

Also, I encourage you to share this newfound knowledge. There are still millions—yes, millions—of people who have no clue about what you have just learned. After all, not too long ago, you were one of them, as was I.

As you work through the book and workbook, you will be asked to write down a variety of goals. At the end of this workbook is a place for you to keep track of each of these vital goals. Keep these goals in front of you—on your refrigerator, bathroom mirror, journal—somewhere they will be at your fingertips, so you see them every day.

Are you ready to apply what you have heard and read and learned? Are you ready to move from a desire to do something to actively committing to it? Let's get started!

Read the Introduction to *Achieving True Wellness in a World of Health Lies*, work through the exercises, and answer the following questions:

For starters, simply write down (yes, stop right now, find a pen or pencil—or your laptop—and write them down!) one or two over-arching goals you hoped to achieve when you committed to this course. Was it just for more knowledge, or did you hope to learn something that would help you accomplish or overcome a specific challenge for you? Write those down.

> ➤ As we move along and as more things become clearer to you—more "ah-has" moments start opening your eyes—you may acquire more or new goals, and that's okay. Write those down too, or even tweak your original goal(s). But for now, write your greatest desire down as a goal, just so you have something to aim for—your "north star," so to speak. You may want

to briefly jump ahead to Chapter 4, under the "Mental Health" section and study how to go about setting goals if this is a practice you have not done in the past.

_____

_____

_____

➤ Has there been a time when you thought you were doing something right for your health, only to find out later (perhaps years later) that it wasn't true? Maybe it was a particular diet or certain foods to eat or not eat. Write out your experience regarding this.

_____

_____

_____

➤ I have no doubt God has you on a journey as He does me. What are some lessons you might have learned along your health journey that you could share with others? Has your "why" originated from one or more of these lessons?

_____

_____

_____

➤ What is a phrase, philosophy, or even a health mandate from an outside entity that you have often thought "that doesn't make sense," but continued to follow the status quo anyway? i.e. "Get your flu shot here for FREE."

_____

_____

_____

➢ Outside of maybe the most commonly discussed internal organs like lungs, heart, brain, and stomach, do you feel confident that you know where all the different parts of your body are and the function(s) they perform?

Yes/No _____

In Chapter 7, we will talk about the liver, adrenals, digestive system, and the gut/brain connection as some core organs or systems of the body. In your own words (don't Google it!), write down what you think some of the functions of these four organs/systems are. If you have no clue, it's okay to write that as your answer. You will know by the end of this course!

_____

_____

_____

_____

_____

➢ What is something you have always "wished for" in regard to your health? Are you willing to make a commitment and do whatever it takes toward achieving it?

_____

_____

_____

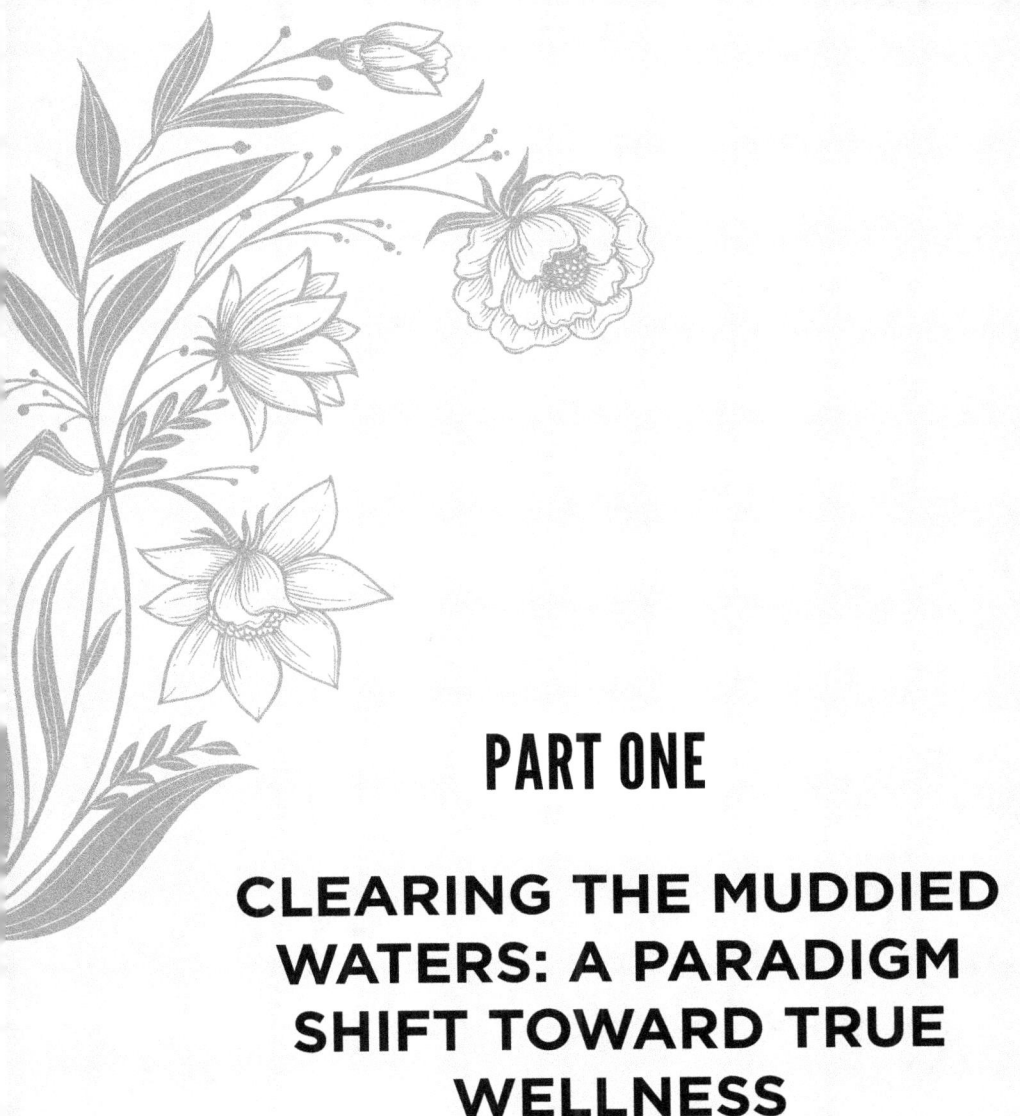

PART ONE

CLEARING THE MUDDIED WATERS: A PARADIGM SHIFT TOWARD TRUE WELLNESS

CHAPTER 1

The Truth About Where Health Comes From

REVIEW

For your first session as a group, spend your review time introducing each participant. Have each member share one thing everybody likely knows about them and one thing they don't.

KEY VERSE

"You made all the delicate, inner parts of my body and knit me together in my mother's womb. Thank you for making me so wonderfully complex! Your workmanship is marvelous—how well I know it. You watched me as I was being formed in utter seclusion, as I was woven together in the dark of the womb. You saw me before I was born. Every day of my life was recorded in your book. Every moment was laid out before a single day had passed." (Psalm 139:13-16 NLT)

VIDEO STREAMING: SESSION 1

INTRODUCTION

As you embark on this course, there will be three foundational keys that will be helpful to keep in mind:

1. You have a unique, divine purpose and reason for being here on this earth.
2. You will need to make a paradigm shift in your thinking as to what true health is.
3. Your health is in your control.

As you proceed through the course, keep coming back to these 3 foundational principles. Without knowing *why* you even get out of bed in the morning, why would you care if you are healthy or not? But you *do* have a reason, and that reason is that you have a purpose. As you progress through the course, you will learn how to discover what that purpose is if you don't already know.

Truly being open to a paradigm shift in your thinking about what wholistic health is will also be vital. I realized this early on, over 20 years ago in fact, as I started teaching others these principles. At times, as I was invited to speak at Lunch & Learns and to civic groups, women's groups, etc., I found myself thinking I needed to eliminate the basic principles of a new paradigm just to shorten the presentation length. But I simply couldn't let go of these vital insights. I felt it essential to bring these principles to light for my audience, otherwise I risked them starting on their newfound journey towards health with their map coordinates off by a degree. You will uncover some of these in chapters two and three. But for now, I invite you to take what you think you know about health and wellness and just set it on a shelf for the duration of this course. Once you are done, I will invite you to take your knowledge back off the shelf and see how it compares to these new insights.

And lastly, take a deep breath, let go of your fears and all that you think you know about health, and simply trust that your health truly is in your control! It's empowering once you start discovering this, and it really is FREEDOM!

One more key component before you move along this new journey: The primary difference between disease management – what most of us think is "health" – and true restoration is: true wholistic health is getting to the "root cause" of any imbalance and then work towards restoring the body to good health utilizing natural approaches.

Keeping these three foundational keys in mind as you move toward your wholistic health restoration will be vital in the success of this journey, not just until you finish the program, but for a lifetime.

Read Chapter 1 of *Achieving True Wellness in a World of Health Lies* and answer the following questions:

> ➤ Do you truly believe that you can have control over your health? Even by just a little bit more than you have now? Why (or why not) and in what way?
>
> _____
>
> _____
>
> _____

Here are some things that God says about "blaming" others and not taking responsibility for our own actions:

Matthew 7:3-5 (ESV) says, "Why do you see the speck that is in your brother's eye, but do not notice the log that is in your own eye? Or how can you say to your brother, 'Let me take the speck out of your eye,' when there is the log in your own eye? You hypocrite, first take the log out of your own eye, and then you will see clearly to take the speck out of your brother's eye."

And Psalm 32:3 (NLT) says, "When I refused to confess my sin, my whole body wasted away, while I groaned all day long."

> ➤ Has there been a time (or two!) in your life when you were sick or diagnosed with something and felt like a victim—like something "got you" that had nothing to do with anything you did? Or perhaps you blamed someone else or someone else's child if you or your child got sick? Write those times down now and revisit that concept as you move through the course. See if your perspective changes as we go along. It's humbling, I know!

_____

_____

_____

➢ Up to this point in your life, do you feel you have been pursuing the disease management approach to what ails you, or is your philosophy more like, "I want to get to the root of what is causing the problem, not just mask it with drugs and/or surgery?"

_____

_____

_____

➢ Take an assessment of your health as a whole—just write down whatever comes to mind that you might like to improve. Assign what you write down to one of the four quadrants of the health pie. For example, it may be a physical issue such as achy joints; an emotional issue where you seem to feel down and depressed for no reason; it could be a mental issue such as spending too much time at work and not enough time with family; and/or perhaps it is spiritual in that you feel distant from God these days. There is no right or wrong place to assign these points of desired improvement—just write them down for now. As we move through the course, continue to assess if the root cause actually lies in the area it is assigned. This will help you recognize where the root is and work toward restoring it to balance.

_____

_____

_____

SUMMARY

- The first thing you must realize is that YOU have a unique divine purpose and reason for being here on this earth.
- The second most important thing is that you will need to make a paradigm shift in your thinking.
- The third thing you need to embrace and have faith in is that your health is in your control—"Health comes from above, down; inside, out."
- There are two main objectives when it comes to following a true wholistic approach to health and wellness:
  1. determine the root cause that is creating the imbalance, and
  2. restore your body to good health using natural approaches.
- Determine whether you want to manage your disease through drugs and surgery, and follow the path of traditional medicine known as disease management, or if you want to uncover the root cause of the problem and restore your body to good health using natural approaches.
- There are four quadrants to the wholistic health pie: mental, emotional, physical, and spiritual.
- There are five pieces to the physical quadrant of the health pie: rest, water, exercise, good nutrition/minus the bad, and good nerve supply.

CHAPTER 2

A Paradigm Shift— What Wellness Is NOT

REVIEW

Discuss what each participant learned, appreciated, and/or applied to their life from last week's session. Any impact on the week's events?

KEY VERSE

"Truth springs from the earth, and righteousness looks down from heaven." (Psalm 85:11 NLT)

VIDEO STREAMING: SESSION 2

INTRODUCTION

I had a conversation with a woman on a flight from Dallas Ft. Worth to Charlotte, NC not too long ago. She shared with me that she worked for a corporate wellness company, and her client was American Airlines. Our flight went by quickly once we engaged in conversation and she learned what I did! But like most conversations with someone new to the wholistic world of health, she would ask me a question, and I would bring her right back to the foundational premise of root cause. In fact, most of her questions went something like this: "What do you think of trace minerals? What do you think of gummy vitamins? What do you think of monk fruit?" And each time I answered her, it gave me a teaching opportunity to instill in her that my perspective wasn't "what do I take" but "what do I do," and I kept reminding her it was about root cause, root cause, root cause.

This is just one of many, many examples of the misunderstanding that people have of what true wholistic health is really all about. That's why this chapter and the next are an exercise in shifting your paradigm from what you *think* health is, and what you've been *told* health is, to what it truly is.

I like to use the analogy of a pilot flying a plane. Before the pilot leaves the runway, he or she needs to have their map coordinates set so that they end up where they intend. They set their starting point as one coordinate, and they set their final destination as another coordinate. They may even have multiple coordinates set in between to be sure they arrive at their final destination in the timeliest way possible.

Your objective with your health is the same way, and the truths about health and wellness are your correct coordinates – if in fact that is what you are aiming for. But the misperceptions about what wellness is *not* and what wellness *is* are like your wrong or correct coordinates. That's why it's important we start here – with the correct coordinates, so that you end up where you want to be – in a place of true understanding of wholistic health and wellness, so that you might live in a place of total health and wellness. Are you ready to get on the plane and pursue the course of optimal health and healing? Then get ready to take off!

Read Chapter 2 of *Achieving True Wellness in a World of Health Lies* and answer the following questions:

These next questions are to help you take an honest assessment of your thought process regarding the truth about health and wellness. Don't beat yourself up for where you are right now, but certainly break down any pride that might keep you from being totally honest with yourself—it's okay! If you really desire to make changes to your health, you need to be honest about where you currently are so you can measure your progress moving forward.

➢ Have you ever been told by a health care practitioner that "everything looks good," and they sent you on your merry way, perhaps with a pill to address your complaint, and yet you still felt lousy? Write what that problem was as well as the outcome of the recommendation or prescription.

_____

_____

_____

➢ On a scale from 1-10 (with 10 being the greatest), how much faith do you put into the annual screenings you may have done to predict that you won't get cancer? Be honest with yourself. A way to tell is if you shrug off doing the things you know you should be doing to take care of your health, and trust that all is well because the screening said so.

_____

_____

_____

SPECTRUM OF HEALTH

100% HEALTH ←—+—+—+—+—⊕—+—+—+—+—→ 99% DISEASE

Estimate where on the "spectrum of health" you think you currently are. Use the halfway point as 50% and break the line down in 10% increments from there: _____%

> ➤ Are you currently taking natural supplements to address symptoms or health conditions you might have been diagnosed with, but you haven't changed any of your lifestyle behaviors, e.g., diet, exercise, etc.?
>
> _____
> _____
> _____

> ➤ Do you know (or even remember) why you decided to take each supplement? Write down the reason you are taking each supplement. If you can't remember, write that down.
>
> _____
> _____
> _____

> ➤ Have you ever made the statement, "It's so expensive to eat healthy?" After reading this chapter, do you still feel the same? Why or why not?
>
> _____
> _____
> _____

> ➤ When you take a look at what you buy to eat at the grocery store, are you truly spending your money on real, nutrient dense food, or does your cart have more of the food-like substances that wouldn't really fit into the definition of real food? What are some real foods you routinely buy, and what are some food-like substances you routinely buy? Write them down.
>
> _____

➤ What food-like substances can you eliminate from your diet and your budget in order to buy something that is more nutrient dense?

➤ If you had the ability to look into your body today and see what kind of materials make up your cells, would they be ready to fall apart from the slightest attack of a foreign substance, or would they be able to stand strong against "the big bad wolf?"

SUMMARY

- There is no magic pill, nor is there even one magic food.
- Wellness is NOT detecting a disease earlier and then starting you on meds earlier.
- Wellness is NOT taking natural supplements for your symptoms.
- The linear path is the path of conventional medicine—symptom here, pain there, take this, problem solved, end of path.
- Don't just mask your symptoms with even a natural product. Get to the root cause of the problem first.
- Wellness does NOT have a shortcut. If it sounds too good to be true, it probably is!
- Wellness is NOT easy. When we start pursuing the path of "easy," we start down a very slippery slope that almost certainly will lead to—at the very least—a waste of time and money, if not a literal detriment to our health.
- Wellness is NOT something your insurance company should pay for.
- "Health" insurance is a misnomer—it is STILL "medical" insurance. If we continually see the word "health" used in the context of conventional medicine (which manages disease and does not restore health), we start thinking it means the same thing—and it doesn't.
- Wellness is NOT too expensive. It's just cheaper to eat food-like substances.

CHAPTER 3

The Paradigm Shift Continued— What Wellness IS

REVIEW

Discuss what each participant learned, appreciated, and/or applied to their life from last week's session. Any impact on the week's events?

KEY VERSE

"Listen to advice and accept instruction, that you may gain wisdom in the future." (Proverbs 19:20 ESV)

VIDEO STREAMING: SESSION 3

INTRODUCTION

As I continue to have conversations with family, friends, total strangers, etc. I realize that there is still a long way to go for the majority of people to truly understand what health really is, and even more so, how to restore it for those who are unhealthy. I am just an average person, and therefore that is who I interact with the most – middle to upper middle-class, average people. Some of these folks are more financially stable than others, some are upper-middle-class, some are lower. Some are highly educated, some not so much. Some young, some older. Regardless of their lot in life, there seems to be a common denominator – they simply have a misunderstanding of how to achieve and maintain optimum health.

I think part of the reason for these misunderstandings is that we are all so bombarded, every which way we look, with the misguided semantics that aim to manipulate, if not confuse us. Probably another reason is that most people don't understand how their body works, where the different parts are, and the function of those parts. To top it off, medical terminology is just flat out baffling. That's why I find it so important to bring these misguided phrases and terminology to light, to help set your feet on the true health path you desire.

In the last session, we talked about just a few of the many semantics and phrases explaining what wellness is NOT. In this chapter, we will take a different perspective on some of these and look at what wellness IS. In a future chapter, we will address four key organs and/or systems of the body to help educate on how the body works and the influence these organs or systems can have on overcoming common symptoms and diseases. Hopefully, by continuing to change your paradigm, you will find your feet on the path of truth as it applies to your health and wellness.

Read Chapter 3 of *Achieving True Wellness in a World of Health Lies* and answer the following questions:

> If you were truly honest with yourself, was there ever a time that you were sick, the doc just gave you "the magic pill," it was easier to "take the quick

fix," and just "keep on doing what you've always done," even though deep down you knew what the root cause was? Write that scenario down—not for anyone else, but as a confession to yourself.

_____
_____
_____

➤ List at least one goal in each area of the four quadrants of the health pie. NOTE: If one of your goals entails improving relations with someone, you can put this under the "emotional" part of the health pie as a social goal.

_____
_____
_____

➤ What is your "why?"

_____
_____
_____

➤ What have you committed to in the past and seen positive results from doing so? Maybe it was a marriage, a job change, or a move to a new town. Or something as simple as spending more time with God. How did it make you feel that you followed through with that commitment? Write it down and include your "why" at the time as a reminder that you can do this when your "why" is great enough.

_____
_____
_____

➢ What are the two main objectives of wholistic health?

_____

_____

_____

➢ Which is your greater desire: to manage your disease (even if you haven't currently been diagnosed with a disease, but you could be) or restore your body to good health/maintain your health? Why?

_____

_____

_____

➢ What small change can you make to overcome a barrier keeping you from achieving a health goal?

_____

_____

_____

➢ Do you take control of your health, or do you just let things happen to your health by thinking, "it will be what it will be?" Write down a time, reflecting on how or why you have made this choice.

_____

_____

_____

➢ As you grab hold of this paradigm shift of what wellness is and/or is not, write out one (or more!) of your own statements from your personal observations:

_____

_____

_____

➢ Wellness is:

_____

_____

_____

➢ Wellness is not:

_____

_____

_____

LET'S GO DEEPER

Now let's see what God might have to say to you about these past two lessons. Write any scripture references that God brings to your heart as you ponder the answers to the following questions:

NOTE: To help in your reflection, you may want to do an internet search such as "what does the Bible say about…"and see what God says to you in what you find.

➢ What is God's Word saying to you about this paradigm shift in your thinking?

_____

_____

_____

➢ What are you feeling challenged by or resistant to in some of the considerations that were just addressed in this chapter or the video? What is God speaking to you about that resistance?

➢ What is one thing that was an "ah-ha" moment for you that you feel you could grab hold of and own?

➢ What is one change you will commit to making as a result of today's lesson?

➢ What do you think God is saying to you about your health and making any changes that might be necessary? Find a scripture that supports what you think He is saying to you and write it out.

➢ Why is your health important to you?

➢ What emotions were triggered for you as each of these truths was brought to light?

➤ What has been a health goal you set for yourself in the past but did not achieve?

CALL TO ACTION

You might be thinking, "What in the heck do the words I use have to do with my health," but I promise you they do. It's a big picture view of what we have been indoctrinated in for years. A paradigm shift in your thinking is an excellent place to start toward making changes. I encourage you to just start paying attention to what you hear, read, and see when it comes to health. Ask yourself, "Is this truly health? Or is this just managing disease?" Make a mental note of it, and even write it down or share your observations with a friend.

SUMMARY

- Wellness IS a life change. If you keep on doing what you've always done, you'll always get what you've always gotten!
- Wellness IS a lifetime commitment. There is a (big) difference between a desire for something and a commitment to it.
- Don't get swept up in the "disease current" because of lack of knowledge, fear, or most importantly, because you think you don't have a choice—you always do.
- Wellness IS bringing the body BACK to good health.
- Many causes can induce the same symptoms.
- Symptoms are simply your body's way of telling you that something is off kilter and to do something about it.
- Suppressing your symptoms with drugs does not fix the problem. You have to change your behavior and get to the root cause of the problem if you want to restore your body to good health.
- Your health IS in your control.
- Wellness IS discipline. No one is going to discipline you when it comes to your health. It's up to you and you alone.
- Wellness IS your insurance.
- Wellness IS common sense simple.
- Wellness IS freedom. Be empowered with this knowledge and these truths. Believe this and start walking it out.

CHAPTER 4

Caring for Your Spiritual, Mental, and Emotional Health

REVIEW

Discuss what each participant learned, appreciated, and/or applied to their life from last week's session. Any impact on the week's events?

KEY VERSE

"I am but a pilgrim here on earth: how I need a map – and your commands are my chart and guide. I long for your instructions more than I can tell."
(Psalm 119:19-20 TLB)

VIDEO STREAMING: SESSION 4

INTRODUCTION

Our health is wholistic – mental, emotional, physical, and spiritual. Our health does not operate in silos, meaning that if we are having problems with a certain body part, it does not function independently of any other area of our body. On the contrary, it throws the entire body out of balance – perhaps not to the degree of the primary organ or system, but it causes a domino effect nonetheless. In addition, when we have a physical health challenge, it also impacts the other three areas of our health – mental, emotional, and spiritual.

Let's use a simple example. If I am having cardiovascular problems, it has now altered my mental health. I'm having to make time to go to doctor appointments, and I'm having to alter my budget to make room for prescription and appointment co-pays, or worse, the cost of a medical procedure. It could limit how I used to spend my social time, therefore impacting my emotional health, not to mention the worry I might be experiencing should my condition get worse, like having a heart attack or stroke. It could even impact my spiritual health – maybe I'm mad at God for allowing something like this to happen to me. This of course is just one example of how one area of our health can and does impact all the others to some degree or another – every time. The examples truly are endless. The fact I'm trying to impress here is that our health, or lack of it, functions as a whole.

In this chapter, we are addressing three of the four components of our health: spiritual, mental, and emotional. We will address the physical part of our health in the next session. I like to start with spiritual health first, as I truly believe it is the core of what could heavily influence the other three areas of our health at any given time.

First, there are three areas of spiritual health:
1. You have a unique divine purpose and reason for being here on this earth. You matter to each and every one of us – we need you, just as you need the rest of us.

2. Learning how to hear God's voice is key to knowing what that purpose is – after all, it is for Him that we are to fulfill that purpose. It's also helpful to hear His voice to know which direction we are to take on any given health decision.
3. Living a spiritually optimal life is dependent on knowing who Jesus is. After all, He is our example on how to live our lives to the fullest. As you study His Word, you will see that He lived wholistically. And if He did, shouldn't we?

In the book and this workbook, I define mental health as addressing our time management, budget, career, goal-setting, and once again, our purpose in life. Our purpose gives us our "why." Why do we even get out of bed in the morning? For example, two primary objections I often hear people voice when it comes to taking care of their health wholistically and naturally are:

- I don't have enough time.
- I don't have enough money.

These are examples of what I mean by mental health.

Our emotional health goes far beyond just positive and negative emotions, although it certainly is that, too. But our emotional health also includes our connection and community with others – our relationships with family, friends, co-workers, church family, our geographic community, etc. Our reproductive hormones have a direct influence on our brain chemicals like dopamine, serotonin, and GABA, mood-regulating hormones. And then there is trauma, especially abuse, but *any* kind certainly has an emotional impact on our wholistic health.

Move forward now by answering the following questions and start assessing where on the spectrum of health your wholistic health might lie.

Read Chapter 4 of *Achieving True Wellness in a World of Health Lies* and answer the following questions:

SPIRITUAL HEALTH

I believe that when you apply the exercise of "How to Hear God's Voice," so much will start coming to light for you. Clarity will begin to emerge. Your faith will grow! As an exercise—and perhaps even a goal or habit moving forward—I invite you to apply these four steps once a day:

1. Quiet Yourself Down
2. Picture Yourself with Jesus
3. Be Open to Spontaneous Thought and Vision
4. Write it Down

Carve out 30 minutes of your day—first thing in the morning, lunch time, before you turn in for the night—and commit to doing this. Even if you can't do it once a day, commit to a certain number of times each week. Simply let God speak to you—yes, He loves it when we come to Him and trust Him with our heart's cries, but He also absolutely adores it when we allow Him to pour out His love onto us. Try it. You won't be sorry you did! It could truly set your feet and your life on a whole new course.

> ➤ Read James 2:14-17. If you were being honest, which direction do you find yourself leaning toward when it comes to your healing and God's part in it: doing all you can do to heal your body but not giving God much room to do His part, or trusting God to heal you while you just keep on doing what you've always done until you are healed? Write down some examples that come to mind to support your answer.
>
> _____
> _____
> _____

> ➤ Would you say you depend more on what God has made for you or on what man has made as it pertains to your health?
>
> _____
> _____
> _____

The Lord then proceeded to tell me why. He said, "I see a dependence on things other than Me, like drugs and medications. I see fear. I see gluttony. I see manip-

ulation, control, and deception by food and drug companies. I see irresponsibility in not caring for the body, My Temple, which I created for each child of Mine. I see abuse of these bodies. This abuse is caused both by the person themselves as well as inflicted by others—this too causes a lack of caring for their Temples. I see a lack of trust in Me to take care of them, not after the fact but instead of. For example, they will eat foods made by man because they are fast, easy, and cheap, rather than eating foods I made for them like fruits, vegetables, grains, and yes, even meats and eggs. They do not slow down long enough to minister to their Temples, they don't slow down to spend time with Me. They are depending on so many other things rather than Me. Food is their god. Poor time management is a real problem. I also see slothfulness, laziness. All of these things hurt My heart and are not My plans for them. They are so ingrained in the so-called comforts of the world that they no longer enjoy the pleasures I made for them. I made my beauty all around them, all things of the earth and sky, land and water, good food from these places, and so much more. Simplicity has been lost—everything is go, go, go."

➢ What part of the above excerpt from the book resonates with you? Why?

_____

_____

_____

➢ Start paying attention to the words you speak this week about yourself and your family. Are they words of life or death? Write down your observations.

_____

_____

_____

➢ Has there been a time when you asked and believed God for something, but your actions ended up being contrary to what you were asking of Him? Journal about this—write that scenario down. If nothing comes to mind, sit down and ask Him—follow the steps on how to hear His voice and ask Him to show you where your actions were not in alignment with your prayers.

➤ What disease seems genetic or hereditary to you and your family that you have either have accepted as your "lot in life" or have refused to control? If you have been "owning" that so-called family gene, commit to breaking off that spiritual stronghold now.

MENTAL HEALTH

➤ Having read this far into the book, what is one goal you are committed to making? What is your "by date" for this goal? What are your action steps?

➤ What is one thing you have stated you can't afford to do as it applies to your health? How much does that one thing cost? Are you committed to doing whatever it takes to be able to afford it, perhaps making a shift in your budget? What can you sacrifice on the financial priority scale to make room for something else that will improve your health? Write it down.

➤ If you could simply die in your sleep when it comes time for you to leave this earth—no diseases, no pain, your body simply finally wears out—how old would you like to be and why?

_____

_____

_____

➤ What is God calling you to do with your time, talent, and resources—right now, today, in this season of your life? Write it down. If you say you don't know, spend time on the four steps of "How to Hear God's Voice" and ask God what His purpose for you is. Write it down.

_____

_____

_____

EMOTIONAL HEALTH

Substances Commonly Recognized to Adversely Affect Our Nervous System Include:

- Industrial chemicals
- Pesticides
- Prescription drugs (the #3 cause of neurotransmitter disease)
- Abused drugs
- Food
- Food additives
- Cosmetic ingredients

➤ Are you, or have you been, routinely exposed to any of these chemicals? If so, list which ones and name them specifically, if you know the name(s). If there are other substances not listed here that you feel could be a problem for your health, list them as well.

_____

_____

_____

➢ Research the various chemicals you are exposed to so you can learn the adverse effects they might have on your health. Write out those adverse effects. Also write out any symptoms you are experiencing that could be caused by these chemicals.

_____

_____

_____

After reading about the symptoms that imbalances in the neurotransmitters can present as, are you experiencing any of these symptoms regularly? Yes/No _____

On a scale from 1-3, with 1 being once every couple of months or less, 2 being once a month or more, and 3 being every week or more, rate the symptoms you are experiencing:

Symptoms of Impaired Acetylcholine Activity:
- Loss of visual and photographic memory _____
- Loss of verbal memory _____
- Memory lapses _____
- Impaired creativity _____
- Diminished comprehension _____
- Difficulty calculating numbers _____
- Difficulty recognizing objects and faces _____
- Slowness of mental responsiveness _____
- Difficulty with directions and spatial orientation _____

Symptoms of Poor Dopamine Activity:

- Inability to self-motivate _____
- Inability to start or finish tasks _____
- Feelings of worthlessness _____
- Feelings of hopelessness _____
- Loss of temper for minor reasons _____
- Inability to handle stress _____
- Anger and aggression while under stress _____
- Desire to isolate oneself from others _____
- Unexplained lack of concern for family and friends _____

Signs of Dopamine Imbalance:

- Iron-deficiency anemia _____
- Depression/lack of motivation _____
- Learning disorders and Attention Deficit Disorder (ADD) _____
- Psychosis _____
- Schizophrenia _____
- Heavy menstrual cycles _____

Symptoms of Impaired Serotonin Activity:

- Loss of pleasure in hobbies and interests _____
- Feelings of inner rage and anger _____
- Feelings of depression _____
- Difficulty finding joy in life pleasures _____
- Depression when it is cloudy or when there is a lack of sunlight _____
- Loss of enthusiasm for favorite activities _____
- Not enjoying favorite foods _____
- Not enjoying friendships and relationships _____
- Unable to fall into deep, restful sleep _____

Symptoms Associated with GABA Imbalances:

- Feelings of anxiousness or panic for no reason   _____
- Feelings of dread   _____
- Feelings of inner tension and inner excitability   _____
- Feelings of being overwhelmed for no reason   _____
- Restless mind   _____
- Hard to turn your mind off when you want to relax   _____
- Disorganized attention   _____
- Worry about things you never thought of before   _____

➢ Based on what you just learned about chemical or emotional stressors, what might you suspect could be causing these symptoms for you?

_____

_____

_____

LET'S GO DEEPER

Write any scripture references that God brings to your heart as you ponder the answers to the following questions:

➢ What is God's Word saying to you about these stressors?

_____

_____

_____

➢ Where are you feeling challenged by or resistant to some of these considerations? What is God speaking to you about that resistance?

_____

_____

_____

➢ What is one thing that was an "ah-ha" moment for you that you feel you could grab hold of and own?

_____

_____

_____

➢ What is one change you will commit to as a result of this week's lesson?

_____

_____

_____

➢ What emotions were triggered for you as each of these truths were brought to light?

_____

_____

_____

CALL TO ACTION

There has been a lot of information in this chapter. In a nutshell, we talked about three of the four quadrants of the health pie—mental, emotional, and spiritual—and then we went into greater detail in each of these areas.

➢ Before locking yourself into searching for only physical roots to a physical health challenge, take into consideration that the root may lie in one of the other 3 areas of your health – spiritual, mental, and/or emotional. Take some time now and think about a physical health challenge you might have, start drilling down past the obvious physical root, and see if the root could be in emotional, spiritual, or mental health. Write down your thoughts.

_____

_____

_____

_____

➤ Take a few minutes and think about the first three quadrants of the health pie and write down one or two goals in each of those areas. They don't need to be overly complicated or time-consuming. Simply write something down to get you started and used to writing down your goals.

_____

_____

_____

➤ Whatever you decide, start writing down some goals outlining what you can COMMIT to doing. Most of all, write down your "why"—why do you want to achieve this goal?

_____

_____

_____

SUMMARY

- Optimum wellness is having your mental, emotional, physical, and spiritual health in balance and functioning.
- All the other pieces of the health pie hinge around our spiritual health. It's the measuring stick. It's where the truth of all the other aspects of our health originates.
- A vital tool for not only our spiritual health, but for our entire health, is to be able to hear God's voice and be confident in that tool.
- Four simple steps to hearing God's voice:
  1. Quiet yourself down.
  2. Picture yourself with Jesus (or Papa God).
  3. Be open to spontaneous thought and vision.
  4. Write down what you hear.
- A good part of whether we succeed in taking control of our health and reversing these chronic degenerative diseases has to do with attitude and the words we speak.
- If we want to make changes to our life, whether mentally, physically, spiritually, or emotionally, we have to have a plan to do so, and it must be written down with an "achieve by" date.
- There are two huge factors that lie within the mental part of our health that can throw the rest of our health out of balance, if not literally into a diseased state: time and money.
- We spend both our time and our money wherever our priorities are.
- Have a written budget and know how many of your dollars are allotted for groceries each week/month.
- Every single one of us has a unique divine reason for being here on this earth.
- YOU are valuable, and we need you. Without YOU, we all fall a little short in our purpose. We need each other for a healthier community and a healthier body of Christ.

CHAPTER 5

Physical Health

REVIEW

Discuss what each participant learned, appreciated, and/or applied to their life from last week's session. Any impact on the week's events?

KEY VERSE

"For you were bought with a price. So glorify God in your body."
(1 Corinthians 6:20 ESV)

VIDEO STREAMING: SESSION 5

INTRODUCTION

Over the years, I have probably had at least one conversation every week with someone who has a total misunderstanding about what true health is. In fact, the physical piece of the wholistic health pie just might be the most misunderstood area of our health, especially as it pertains to how to prevent chronic disease and how to restore the body to good health, using natural approaches. But it's not for the lack of information out there. It's out there — everywhere. The problem lies not in the tools available but in the objective.

In fact, I have come to realize that the core of my personal objective or reason for being here on this earth is to continually reveal the difference between the two approaches: disease management and health restoration—wholistic health. This is why I started off this workbook, the accompanying book, and the online course by impressing on you the need for a paradigm shift in your thinking. One of those shifts is to change your thinking to "it's not what do I take, but what do I do?"

Last session, we addressed three of the four quadrants of our wholistic health — spiritual, mental, and emotional. In this session, we will take a look at physical health. There are 5 foundational pieces to our physical health. It is imperative that you start with these five priorities when addressing your physical health. I promise you, they will go a long way for the majority of the more common chronic diseases out there. Four of these five areas are within your total control. For the fifth one, you will need assistance from a licensed chiropractor. Once you've brought these 5 areas into balance, then and only then should you seek out the assistance of a functional medicine practitioner. We will talk more in Chapter 10 about all the natural disciplines that could fall under this umbrella of functional medicine, but you need to take charge of your health first. Otherwise, they are simply going to instruct you to do the same things I have, and you may as well save yourself some time and money by getting a jump on these five areas before seeking the assistance of a professional. A lot of this work is in your capable hands.

The five areas are:

Rest

Adults need 8-9 hours of quality sleep every night. Children need at least 10. The body does its best healing and repairing between 10:00 at night and midnight. And the only time the body can naturally regenerate itself is when we are sleeping.

Water

There are 4 organs and/or systems of the body utilized by the body to eliminate its waste and toxins. 50% of the body's waste should be eliminated through the kidneys,. 25% through the skin, 23% through the lungs, and 2% through the colon. But the key to each of these organs or systems is: they all need enough water to do so. Otherwise, the toxins stay in our bodies, causing inflammation, which leads to disease.

Exercise

While exercise is helpful to burn calories, the main reason we all think of when we hear "exercise," we also know it's good for our cardiovascular health. But it goes way beyond that. Even conventional medicine will say exercise is a better antidepressant than a medication is. Exercise helps move the toxins out of the body, in part through our lungs and skin. Exercise boosts our metabolism, which plays a vital role in all functions of our body – digestion, cardiovascular health, sleep regulation, and simply slowing down the aging process in general.

Good Nutrition

This area is huge and probably the most misunderstood, for both its harm and its benefits. We are either putting something of value into our mouths and our bodies, or something *not* of value. We literally are what we eat. Whatever we put into our mouths becomes the building block for the next cells that need to be formed. Old cells die every day, and new ones are made every day. And it is what we feed our body that becomes the next cells. Would you want to live in a house built of poor quality construction materials or strong, durable, long-lasting materials? Our body houses our life. But you know what else it houses? The Most High Living God, the One Who created your body and assigned it to you to begin with, literally resides on the inside of you. Let that sink in for a minute. If you knew Jesus was coming for a visit, would you not want your home to look the best it ever had? Well, knock, knock – He's already there!

Good Nerve Supply

This is the fifth piece of the physical part of the health pie, the one that requires assistance from a licensed chiropractor. Now, you might be saying to yourself, "I don't have back or neck pain." Well, guess what? That is another deception! Chiropractic care is not just about back and neck pain. It's about restoring good nerve supply to your body. Think of your nervous system as the electrical wiring in your house. One little short, and all kinds of things aren't working right. Your nervous system works the same way. Every cell, tissue, organ, and system of the body needs a healthy nerve supply, every minute of every day. But when there is interference with the nervous system, at the spinal column, that interferes with the optimal function of your body.

Read Chapter 5 of *Achieving True Wellness in a World of Health Lies* for a deeper understanding of each of these five areas of physical health, and then answer the following questions:

> ➤ On a scale from 1-10, on average over one month, how well would you say you sleep?
>
> How many hours a night do you sleep?
>
> _____
> _____
> _____
>
> ➤ What time do you fall asleep (not simply get into bed), and what time do you get out of bed for the day?
>
> _____

➢ Unless you have rated your sleep as a consistent 10, please answer the following questions:

Based on the suggestions listed in this chapter on sleep or other ideas you have heard, what can you do to improve your sleep?

➢ What is your goal for sleep? What are your action steps to fulfill this goal? Write it down in a S.M.A.R.T. goal format, making it specific, measurable, achievable, relevant, and timely.

➢ On average, how much water do you drink a day? (Do not include all liquids, only water.) How much do you currently weigh? Divide your body weight in half (e.g., if you weigh 150 pounds, half your body weight would be 75 pounds). Now convert that number from pounds into ounces. This is your new goal for water consumption! Write it down.

TAKE AN INVENTORY TO GET YOU STARTED

➢ What is exercise to you?

_____

_____

_____

➢ What might keep you from exercising—time, location, dislike, etc.?

_____

_____

_____

➢ How can you overcome these barriers?

_____

_____

_____

➢ Are you currently on a REGULAR exercise program?

Yes_____   No_____

_____

_____

_____

➢ How often do you exercise?

_____

_____

_____

➢ For how long?

_____

_____

_____

➢ What kind of exercise are you doing or would you like to do?

_____

_____

_____

➢ What do you think are the benefits of exercise to you?

_____

_____

_____

➢ Before reading what a chiropractor does, what did you think they did?

_____

_____

_____

➢ If you've been to a chiropractor in the past, what was your reason for going? How long did you go? Did they use the word "subluxation?" If so, did they explain to you the definition of it? Write down what you now know a chiropractor does so that you can tell others what they do.

_____

_____

_____

➢ If you aren't currently under chiropractic care, do you now find the value in going, even if you don't have back or neck pain? Why or why not?

_____

_____

_____

➤ List all the different diet plans you have followed over the years. Include what your reason was for doing so and whether it worked for you. Have you been able to maintain whatever that goal was?

_____

_____

_____

➤ How often do you eat fast food per day/week/month/year?

_____

_____

_____

Keep a log of all the foods you consume for an entire week, including snacks (see the food log at the back of this workbook). Also include foods you might have eaten out—whether dining out, a networking event, a breakfast meeting, or having dinner at a friend's house. Don't feel you need to suddenly "eat healthy." This log is for your eyes and your eyes alone (unless you want to be held accountable by someone else). Beside each food, mark an "I" (for inflammatory) or an "N" (for non-inflammatory). This exercise is meant to bring true awareness of what you eat in a week and where you consume those foods.

Keep a record of how much sugar you eat and the form it is in—processed sugar, honey, agave nectar, stevia, artificial sweeteners, etc.—for one week. Total up your sugar intake in teaspoons. Write that number here: _____.

NOTE: 4 grams of sugar = roughly 1 teaspoon.

Here are some symptoms of sugar imbalances:

(Circle any of the symptoms you experience regularly.)

Symptoms of Hypoglycemia (low blood sugar):
- Having increased energy after meals
- Cravings for sweets between meals
- Irritability when meals are missed

- Dependency on coffee and sugar for energy
- Becoming lightheaded if meals are missed
- Eating to relieve fatigue
- Feeling shaky, jittery, or tremulous
- Feeling agitated and nervous
- Becoming easily upset
- Poor memory, forgetfulness
- Blurred vision

Symptoms of Insulin Resistance:
- Fatigue after meals
- General fatigue
- Constant hunger
- Craving sweets or relieved by eating them
- Must have sweets after meals
- Waist girth equal to or larger than hip girth
- Frequent urination
- Increased appetite and thirst
- Difficulty losing weight
- Migrating aches and pains

Symptoms of sugar hangover:
- Fuzzy thinking or foggy mind
- Fatigue or sleepiness after meals
- Gas, bloating, or extended stomach after meals
- Headache
- Joint pain
- Constipation
- Diarrhea

- Skin problems
- Allergy symptoms

Emotional Symptoms of Sugar Hangover:
- Mood swings like emotional highs and lows (anger, sadness, lack of willpower, depression, etc.)
- Feelings similar to having too much alcohol—and there's a reason for that

Physical Effects of Sugar Hangover:
- Kidneys are affected
- Liver is compromised
- Stomach issues
- Small intestines are not functioning optimally
- Dehydration
- Electrolyte imbalances
- Gastrointestinal disturbances
- Sleep disruption

➤ When you think about eating an all (or 80%) raw food diet, what challenges might come to mind? Write them down. Now, beside them, write some ways you can overcome those challenges.

_____
_____
_____
_____

LET'S GO DEEPER

Write any scripture references that God brings to your heart as you ponder the answers to the following questions:

➤ What are you feeling challenged by or resistant to in some of the considerations in this lesson? What is God speaking to you about that resistance?

_____
_____
_____

➤ What is one thing that was an "ah-ha" moment for you that, with God's help, you feel you could grab hold of and take ownership of?

_____
_____
_____

➤ What is one change you feel God prompting you to commit to as a result of this week's lesson?

_____
_____
_____

➤ What emotions were triggered for you as each of these truths was brought to light?

_____
_____
_____

CALL TO ACTION

We broke down the physical part of the health pie into greater detail—rest, water, exercise, good nutrition, and good nerve supply.

➤ Take a few minutes and think about the physical part of the health pie. Write down one or two goals in this particular area of your health. They don't need to be overly complicated or time-consuming. Simply write something down to get you started and get used to writing down your goals.

___

➤ You may want to look at the five pieces of the physical quadrant and write a goal or two for each of those areas, such as increasing your water intake, starting an exercise plan, or eliminating fast food, fried foods, packaged/processed foods and sugar. Maybe that is too much at once. If so, start first with eliminating sugar or perhaps cow's milk! You may feel 100% better just by doing that!

___

Whatever you decide, start writing down some goals outlining what you can COMMIT to doing. Most of all, write down your "why"—why do you want to achieve this goal?

SUMMARY

- Lack of sleep has a direct negative impact on the majority of chronic degenerative diseases.

- There are four main organs or systems the body uses to rid itself of waste and toxins. 50% of the body's waste should be eliminated through the kidneys. 25% percent should be eliminated through the skin, 23% through the lungs, and 2% through the colon. All four of these mechanisms need water for the waste and toxins to come out of the body.

- Check out your county Parks and Recreation website or the local Chamber of Commerce and Visitor Bureau for a wealth of enjoyable ideas and opportunities for you to exercise.

- A subluxation is when the bones in our back or neck, called vertebrae, are misaligned. Just a millimeter of shift is all it takes, and they can stay stuck or locked in that position, putting pressure on the spinal nerves that pass between the bones and causing a lowered state of health. Initially, you most likely won't even feel this pressure.

CHAPTER 6

Inflammatory versus Non-Inflammatory Foods

REVIEW

Discuss what each participant learned, appreciated, and/or applied to their life from last week's session. Any impact on the week's events?

KEY VERSE

"And God said, "Behold, I have given you every plant yielding seed that is on the face of all the earth, and every tree with seed in its fruit. You shall have them for food."
(Genesis 1:29 ESV)

VIDEO STREAMING: SESSION 6

INTRODUCTION

The common denominator of all chronic degenerative diseases is inflammation, and there are four interchangeable words when it comes to inflammation and our health:

stress = inflammation = acidic (systemic pH) = toxic

I elaborate more on all of these in the book and video, but for now, let's focus on two: stress = inflammation.

If I asked you for some examples of stress, you would most likely start throwing out topics like work, finances, family, relationships, spouse, and even health. And those *are* all examples of stress. But they are specifically examples of mental/emotional stress. There are two other categories of stress that we tend to overlook: physical and chemical. One example of physical stress could be over-exercising (don't get excited, this is not to be used as permission to not exercise!). The key word here is "over" exercising. I backpack, and this is no doubt stressful to the physical body. While I used to hike 15-18 miles a day in my 50s, and I have sensed backed off on the mileage a bit, it is still physical stress to the body. Even though I've backed down on the mileage, I have also aged 10 years! Breaking a leg, having surgery, and not sleeping well or enough are other examples of physical stress to the body. And then there are chemical stresses to the body: the foods we eat, the air we breathe, and the water we drink are just a few examples. Medications, illicit drug use, excessive alcohol consumption, cigarettes – these are also examples of chemical stresses.

Now, replace all of these examples of stress with the word "inflammation," and you have a broad brush painted picture of the root cause of all our chronic degenerative diseases! I have included here in the workbook a short-list of inflammatory foods and a short-list of non-inflammatory foods to help you get started on measuring some of the chemical stresses you might be subjecting your mind and body to, as well as examples of healing foods – foods that can be your medicine.

Read Chapter 6 of *Achieving True Wellness in a World of Health Lies* and answer the following questions:

It's not about the calories—it's about the right nutrients.

Write out the four words that are interchangeable:

1. _____
2. _____
3. _____
4. _____

Remember the four interchangeable words when answering these:

List at least three mental/emotional stressors you are either currently experiencing or have experienced over the past year. Keep in mind, mental/emotional stressors can also be "good" things, e.g., getting married, buying a new home, having a baby, etc.

1. _____
2. _____
3. _____
4. _____
5. _____

List at least three physical stressors your body has experienced over the past year.

1. _____
2. _____
3. _____
4. _____
5. _____

List at least three chemical stressors your body is exposed to regularly, including the air you breathe, the water you drink, the foods you eat, and any medications you take.

1. _____
2. _____

3. _____
4. _____
5. _____

Inflammatory Foods

- Fast food
- Fried foods
- PACKAGED and PROCESSED foods (this list of foods is huge)
- Sugars
- Animal products
- Grains

Non-Inflammatory Foods

- Fruits
- Vegetables
- Nuts and seeds
- Good fats (like avocados, flax seed, olive oil, coconut oil – LOVE coconut oil!)
- Water

Anything that has a food label on it and comes in a "package" is a packaged food.

4 grams of sugar = roughly 1 teaspoon. Think about this measurement every time you look at how much sugar is in a product (and you should look every time).

LET'S GO DEEPER

Write any scripture references that God brings to your heart as you ponder the answers to the following questions:

➤ Which of the inflammatory foods do you feel you could be addicted to?
_____
_____
_____

➤ What is God's Word saying to you about this category of food? Is He perhaps asking you to surrender it to Him? What else might he be saying?
_____
_____
_____

➤ Where are you feeling challenged by or resistant to some of these considerations? What is God speaking to you about that resistance?
_____
_____
_____

➤ What is one thing that was an "ah-ha" moment for you that you feel you could grab hold of and own?
_____
_____
_____

➤ What is one change you will commit to as a result of today's lesson?
_____
_____
_____

➢ What emotions were triggered for you as each of these truths was brought to light?

_____
_____
_____

➢ Why do you think it would be important to God that you commit to making a change in your health in this area?

_____
_____
_____

CALL TO ACTION

Choose one category from the inflammatory foods list and totally eliminate it. If you already don't eat much fast food, then start there if you must, for a week. Check it off your goals list as a win, and move on to the next least invasive food-like substance you consume. Eliminate it for a period of time and keep working your way off the inflammatory foods list.

As you eliminate inflammatory foods, your meals might start getting smaller, so add a non-inflammatory food to your plate to replace a category of food you have eliminated. Start exchanging bad for good.

SUMMARY

- Four words are interchangeable: stress, inflammation, acidic pH, and toxic.
- There are 3 types of stressors: mental/emotional, physical, and chemical.
- Some examples of chemical stressors could be the air you breathe, the water you drink, medications/drugs you take, and the food-like substances you eat.
- The short list of inflammatory foods are: fast food, fried food, packaged/processed foods, and sugars. Also conventionally raised/grown animal products and grains.
- The short list of non-inflammatory foods are: fruits, vegetables, nuts & seeds, good fats, and water.

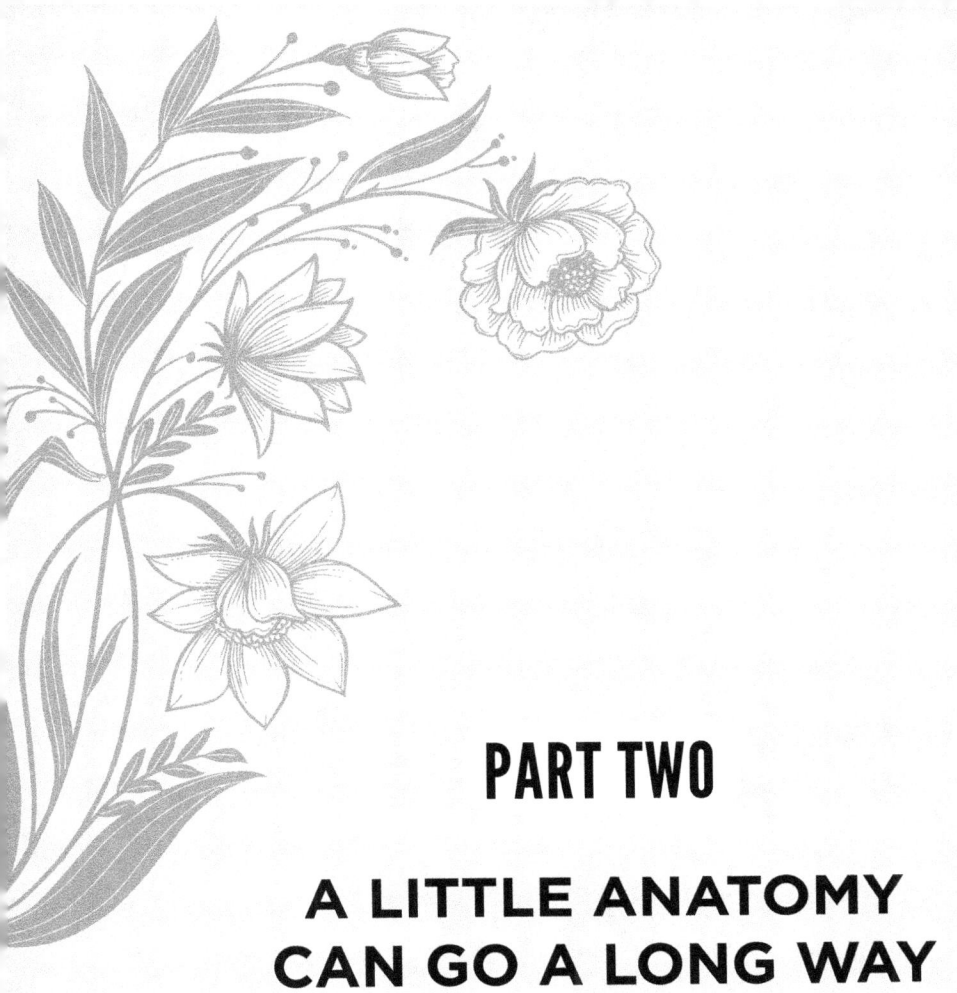

PART TWO

A LITTLE ANATOMY CAN GO A LONG WAY

CHAPTER 7

Four Organs and Systems of the Body That Can Extend Your Health!

REVIEW

Discuss what each participant learned, appreciated, and/or applied to their life from last week's session. Any impact on the week's events?

KEY VERSE

"For just as in one [physical] body we have many parts, and these parts do not all have the same function or special use, so we, who are many, are [nevertheless just] one body in Christ, and individually [we are] parts one of another [mutually dependent on each other]." (Romans 12:4-5 AMP)

VIDEO STREAMING: SESSION 7

INTRODUCTION

Traditional medicine has become so specialized. What do I mean by that? There is now a medical practitioner specializing in almost every specific organ or system of the body. If you were to look in the handbook you probably received when you enrolled in an insurance plan, you would probably find dozens of different types of specialties related to the symptom that ails you. For example, I just looked at providers on my online healthcare portal and typed in "ear, nose, and throat." There were 9 different subspecialties just under this one specialty! The overarching specialty for all traditional medicine is disease management, and each specialist works in their own silo.

Let me share a personal experience to demonstrate what I mean. I currently see a hematologist, a blood cancer specialist within the specialty field of oncology. I take medication for a gene mutation in the bone marrow that causes high blood platelets. While the medication is a "tried and true" medication that has been around a long time, it is not exempt from being able to cause adverse side effects, effects to the liver and kidneys in particular. While I have only been on this medication for a short time, I keep an eye on my liver and kidney markers. If either of those organs start to have problems because of the medication, the hematologist is not prepared, lacks the knowledge, and doesn't even have the time to address these concerns for me. He would have to refer me to a kidney specialist or a hepatology specialist. And what's worse is he is not overly concerned about labs being off until they reach a diseased range – a "wait and see" approach. Functional medicine operates in a whole different paradigm. When we analyze bloodwork, we look at it wholistically – taking into consideration all the markers and how they work together. We don't take a "wait and see" approach. We start looking for the root cause of the various inter-connected markers that are out of functional range, or subclinical if you will, which is far earlier than a disease range.

Over my years as a functional medicine practitioner, time and time again what I have found is there are 4 organs and/or systems of the body that we could tie as the root cause to the majority of the most common chronic diseases and imbalances to. Those are:

- Adrenals
- Liver
- Digestive System
- And the Gut/Brain connection

I go into much greater detail in the book as to the vital role of each of these organs and/or systems and how the root of the many common chronic diseases can be traced back to them. In the book, I also bring your attention to one more organ, the largest organ of our body, in fact, and that is the skin. Not so much because we can tie the majority of chronic disease back to skin being the root issue, but because it is extremely overlooked regarding proper care of it—what we put on it, like dental products, skin care products, hair products, body soaps, makeup, hair dyes, and the list goes on and on. In fact, I recently bit the bullet and decided to let my natural hair color present itself for the first time in 50 years! As you can probably guess, that natural color is now a crowning head of gray, but for 50 years, I put highly toxic chemicals on my hair and head that easily entered my body.

Read Chapter 7 of *Achieving True Wellness in a World of Health Lies* and answer the following questions:

To start your new health program, I suggest starting with a quality liver detox.

To do a liver detox, I recommend either ordering through my professional link for the Biotics Nutriclear 15-day detox: https://us.fullscript.com/welcome/jmckool/store-start (my highest recommendation). If that is out of your comfort area cost-wise, my second best recommendation would be the 30-day Liver Detox by Renew Life: https://www.renewlife.com/products/liver-detox-cleansing-formula-30-day-program-rn15525.

- How frequently do you get sick, even with a cold? If it's more than once a year, your immune system is most likely compromised in some way.

- Do you experience heartburn or acid reflux? Yes/No _____

- Are you taking antacids—either over the counter or prescription? Yes/No _____

- Have you been diagnosed with osteopenia or osteoporosis? Yes/No _____

- Have you been told that you are low in calcium, magnesium, or Vitamin D? Yes/No _____

- Or are you experiencing symptoms related to a deficiency in any or all of these vitamins and/or minerals? Yes/No _____

- How has your protocol been working for you?

_____

_____

If all it has been doing is minimizing your symptoms, but nothing else, consider supplementing with hydrochloric acid (HCl).

CAUTION: If you have been diagnosed with stomach ulcers or suspect that you might have stomach ulcers, do NOT take hydrochloric acid.

NOTE: To take both an antacid AND HCl would be counterproductive to both. They basically cancel each other out. Consider talking with your prescribing physician about eliminating the medicine and trying HCl. See if that might make a difference with your symptoms as well as your calcium, magnesium, and/or vitamin D levels.

- Are you experiencing a multitude of symptoms, no matter how minor, but nothing seems to resolve the problem? Yes/No _____

- Have you been diagnosed or suspect that you have an autoimmune condition? Yes/No _____

- Have you ever had a hidden food sensitivity test done? Yes/No _____

- Are you experiencing some digestive imbalances (even if they are minor)? Yes/No _____

Consider seeking out a healthcare practitioner who can order a hidden food sensitivity test for you, and consider consuming a non-inflammatory diet if you are not already doing so.

- How many ounces of water do you drink on average per day? _____

- Do you experience constipation? Yes/No _____

If you are sitting on the toilet longer than a minute or two to relieve your bowels, and/or if you are not having at least one bowel movement a day, you most likely are experiencing constipation to some degree. If you don't have daily bowel movements, you absolutely are not only constipated, but your body has inflammation and is toxic.

If you are not drinking half of your body weight in ounces of water each day, commit to doing so. Write out a goal of consuming the minimum amount of water a day that you need, then create a plan to achieve that goal and stick with it.

The daily minimum number of ounces of water needed is equivalent to half your body weight. For example, a person weighing 150 pounds needs 75 ounces of water daily.

To recap, here are some foundational supplements to assist the digestive system in functioning optimally: HCl for the stomach, a good digestive enzyme for the small intestine, and a quality probiotic for the colon. The HCl and digestive enzymes should only be taken with meals. The best time to take the probiotic is at bedtime, once the digestive system has done its work for the day.

- ➤ Whether you are closer to the left end of the spectrum of health or have been diagnosed with a disease, in which of the four organs/systems do you think your root cause might lie, and why?

_____

_____

_____

LET'S GO DEEPER

Write any scripture references that God brings to your heart as you ponder the answers to the following questions:

➤ Which area of the body resonates the most with you regarding needing your focus for healing?

_____
_____
_____

➤ What is God's Word saying to you about any one of these areas of the body?

_____
_____
_____

➤ Where are you feeling challenged by or resistant to some of these considerations? What is God speaking to you about that resistance?

_____
_____
_____

➤ What is one thing that was an "ah-ha" moment for you that you feel you could grab hold of and own?

_____
_____
_____

➤ What is one change you will commit to as a result of today's lesson?

_____

➢ What emotions were triggered for you as each of these truths was brought to light?

➢ Why do you think it would be important to God that you commit to making a change in your health?

CALL TO ACTION

Start taking a probiotic at bedtime. Start tonight!

Take an inventory of all your personal care items, as well as detergents and cleaning products. Look at the ingredients in them, just as you would your food. Start doing research on these brands as well. There are a variety of websites that can help you do this. Also see the "Suggested Reading and Resources" section at the end of the book. Gradually exchange any "dirty ingredient" products with clean ingredient ones.

I encourage you to start healing. Perhaps you start with a liver detox or start taking some supplements for your digestive health. Maybe you do an assessment to the stressors in your life—chemical, mental/emotional, and physical. How can you start reducing that stress? Remember that stress, inflammation, acidic pH, and toxicity are interchangeable—if one is there, the others are there. Minimize the stress, and you will minimize the inflammation.

Set a goal and some action steps to tackle the area you want to heal first. One step at a time—even baby steps are steps in the right direction.

And remember: your health IS in your control!

SUMMARY

- There are four organs or systems of the body (called the "heavy hitters") that the majority of our chronic degenerative imbalances and diseases can be traced back to. At least one of them is your root cause.
- The liver has over 500 functions, and those are only the ones we know of.
- The main organs of the digestive system are the stomach, small intestine, and large intestine (also known as the colon). Other organs that contribute greatly to the digestive process are the gallbladder, liver, and pancreas. The appendix has a role to play as well.
- Here are some foundational supplements to assist the digestive system in functioning optimally: HCl for the stomach, a good digestive enzyme for the small intestine, and a quality probiotic for the colon. The HCl and digestive enzymes should only be taken with meals, and the best time to take the probiotic is at bedtime, once the digestive system has done its work for the day.
- You can still benefit from the gallbladder flush discussed in this chapter even if your gallbladder has been removed. In most cases, what is known as the "biliary tree"—the various ducts that go to the gallbladder—is still there. Stones and sludge can accumulate here as well.
- Remember, 70 % of the immune system is in the gut. The digestive system is now referred to as the body's "second brain." The digestive system actually has its own nervous system, called the enteric nervous system, and communicates with the brain through the phrenic nerve. There certainly is direct communication and influence from the gut to the brain and the brain to the gut. If the digestive system is unhealthy, there is no question that the brain is as well.
- The skin has the ability to absorb anything we put on it, good or bad.

CHAPTER 8

The Connection Between Trauma & Addiction "Which Came First, The Chicken or The Egg?" (Stress or Addiction?)

REVIEW

Discuss what each participant learned, appreciated, and/or applied to their life from last week's session. Any impact on the week's events?

KEY VERSE

"The Spirit of the Lord GOD is upon me; because the LORD hath anointed me to preach good tidings unto the meek; he hath sent me to bind up the brokenhearted, to proclaim liberty to the captives, and the opening of the prison to them that are bound;"
(Isaiah 61:1 NKJ)

VIDEO STREAMING: SESSION 8

INTRODUCTION

For about six years, I worked as the development director for a non-profit women's ministry. We served women who were walking out their recovery as well as women who were experiencing homelessness. What I learned fairly quickly in my time there was that abuse, addiction, homelessness, and mental health challenges quite often go hand in hand. Every scenario was different, and the challenge was trying to discern what came "first," the addiction, homelessness, or mental health challenges? In other words, "What came first, the chicken or the egg?" But here is the thing: a common denominator with each one of these is quite often abuse, and abuse is trauma, and trauma equals stress, and stress equals inflammation.

During my time there, I gave a lot of presentations on behalf of the ministry to women's church groups. The groups often consisted of women in their 60s, 70s, and 80s. And almost always, there was at least one woman in that group, if not multiple, who had experienced abuse in their younger years. As I shared with them about the women in the recovery program experiencing abuse, I could see some of the women lowering their eyes, their minds taking off to a place many years before – reflecting on their own suppressed trauma. Occasionally, I would have a lady come up to me afterward and share her story of abuse with me. In most cases, these women's lives were spared the path of addiction, but unless the pain and trauma were addressed at some point, they were still carrying around a very heavy burden of guilt and shame. Now, I was not there to speak with them about wholistic health and wellness, but I would love to have had the opportunity to visit with them longer to see if they were experiencing any kind of chronic health challenges and to share with them not to overlook the connection between their current physical health challenges and the trauma they experienced.

Our society is filled with so many stories of abuse and trauma. Not just women, but men as well. Quite often this abuse and trauma initially occurred in childhood, a lot of the time at the hands of the one who was to be the protector – a mother, father, other relative, pastor, teacher, scout leader, community service member, and the list goes on. Trauma certainly lies in the emotional part of the health pie, but make no mistake, it has tremendous adverse effects on physical and spiritual health as well. I truly believe that this is a root cause of a lot of the tremendous gender confusion, school shootings, and suicides among young people, not to mention their poor eating habits, lack of purpose and motivation, and so much more. The subject of the impacts of trauma on the mind and body is too often overlooked when it comes to the health decline of our young people, the general population, and our communities as a whole.

Read Chapter 8 of *Achieving True Wellness in a World of Health Lies* and do the following exercises:

(You may want to grab a pen and paper, or you can use your computer for these exercises to give yourself plenty of room to write.)

Ask yourself, "What am I addicted to?" Have you experienced any traumas, especially as a child? A word of caution and encouragement here: what you might not think of as a trauma probably was. Don't dismiss the harmful things that have happened in your life—even if it was no one's fault. Perhaps your house caught on fire, you were in a bad car accident, you had a very frightful scare, or maybe a dog attacked you as a child. The possibilities could be endless. Give thought to these events and address them. Perhaps seek some counseling or, at the very least, share your trauma with a trusted friend, family member, or spouse. But don't underestimate the influence that this or multiple traumas can have on the challenges you may face in overcoming your health problems.

Sit for a moment, reflecting on your life. Think of your childhood, as far back as you can remember. Take time examining your life from all angles—your home life, school life, friends, adversaries, good memories, and hard-to-face memories. Block it off by decades, starting with 0-10 years old, then 11-20 years old, and so on, to help you break down your reflection time into smaller pieces. You may even want to journal about what might have been going on in your family's lives before you were born, especially when you were in utero.

Did traumatic events take place in any of these blocks of time? Write them down. Don't rush this—write whatever comes to your mind without analyzing whether an event was traumatic or not. Just write—as much as you want or need. This is for you and you alone.

Perhaps there are some situations that your memory won't even allow you to recall, and that's okay. Write down these more significant times in your life (remember, if it feels significant to you, it WAS significant—even if someone else doesn't think so). Make a note, especially of those things that seem to remain on the surface.

For example, there was a time in my grade school years when, in my mind, every classmate hated me. They ostracized me, they talked about me, they were verbally mean to me, for what seemed like weeks. Now, was it really every single classmate or just a few? Was it really for weeks, or was it more like a couple of days? It doesn't matter. I can't even remember the details, but this scenario comes up quite often when I give attention to what I might not like about myself. Or why don't I trust people? For me, this must have been some kind of trauma. For someone else? They might think, "Lady, that's child's play, you don't have any idea what trauma is." And they are probably right—regardless, it was traumatic to me.

Face the traumas you may have experienced, acknowledge them, and give grace to yourself for the negative impacts they may have had—and possibly still have—on your life. If you need to, talk with a licensed counselor about it. Don't allow unresolved trauma to take hold of your life any longer than it already has. Remember: trauma = stress, stress = inflammation, and inflammation is the common denominator of all chronic degenerative diseases. Get to the root and heal from it.

LET'S GO DEEPER

Write any scripture references that God brings to your heart as you ponder the answers to the following questions:

> ➢ Now that you have a better understanding of what trauma is, sit with Papa God and ask Him to show you any hurts that might be deep in your heart. What is He showing you, and what is He saying to you about the root cause of this pain? Don't minimize whatever He brings to mind, just follow Him, and let Him show you ways it might be affecting your overall health. Write down all that He is saying and/or showing you.

➢ What is God's Word saying to you about what He is revealing in your heart? Write a healing scripture to overcome the hurt.

➢ Where are you feeling challenged by or resistant to what He might be showing you? What is God speaking to you about that resistance? Is there anyone you may need to forgive for what He is showing you – another person, God, yourself?

➢ What is one thing that was an "ah-ha" moment for you that you feel you could grab hold of and own?

➢ What is one change you will commit to moving forward as a result of today's lesson?

➢ What emotions were triggered for you as each of these truths was brought to light?

_____
_____
_____

➢ Why do you think it would be important to God that you commit to making a change in your overall health as it pertains to what He has revealed to you?

_____
_____
_____

CALL TO ACTION

Have empathy and grace either for yourself or for others who might be walking in addiction, mental health challenges, or even walking out their recovery. Understand that their lives are wholistic too, whether out of balance or in balance, and we are all on a journey. Meet them (or even yourself) where they/you currently are.

SUMMARY

- Trauma=Stress, and Stress=Inflammation=Toxic. And drugs—whether prescription or street drugs—are very toxic to the body. In the most basic sense, are you starting to see the common denominators here? These words are interchangeable. Things like mental, emotional, physical, verbal, and sexual abuse are 100% trauma *and* 100% stress.

- Make no mistake: abuse is trauma. Post-Traumatic Stress Disorder can lead to substance abuse, psychiatric issues, physical pain, sleep problems, cognitive symptoms, medical conditions, relationship problems, etc.

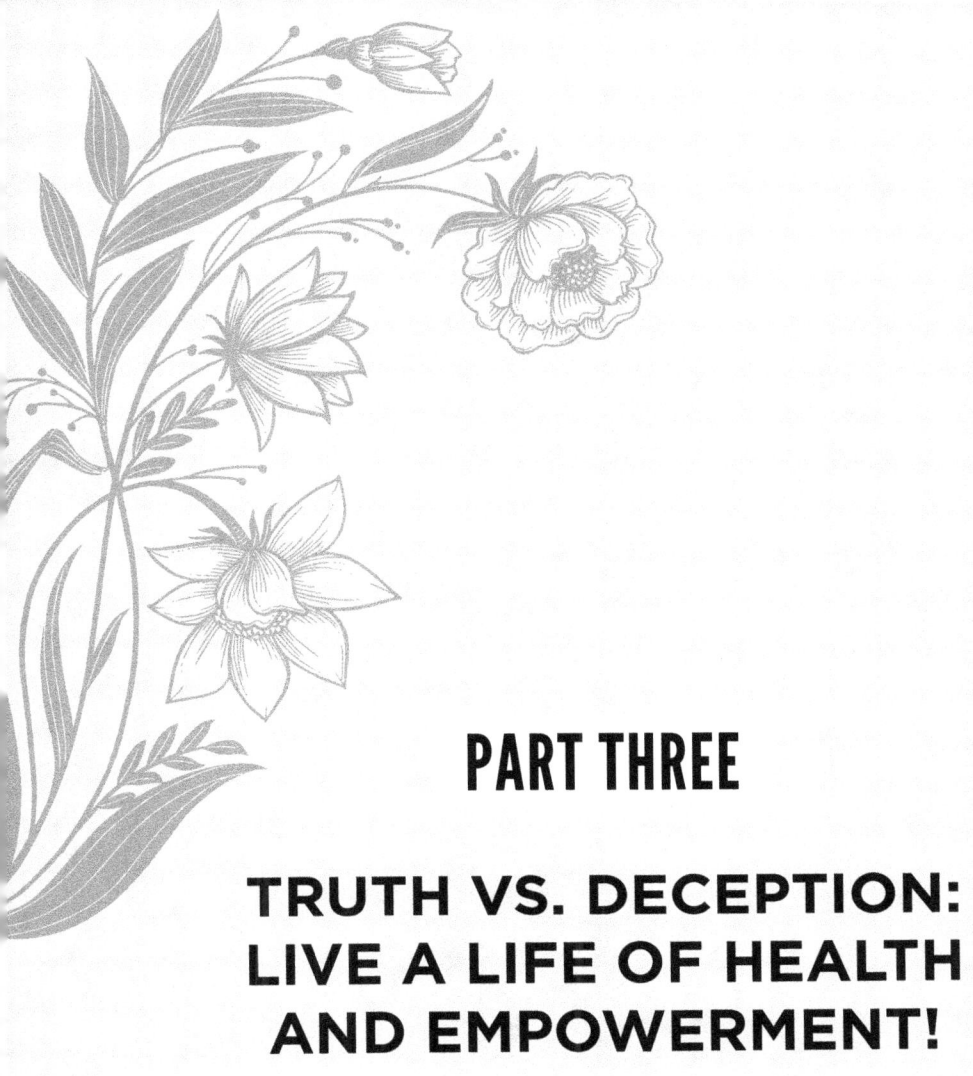

PART THREE

TRUTH VS. DECEPTION: LIVE A LIFE OF HEALTH AND EMPOWERMENT!

CHAPTER 9

The Truths—Open Your Eyes and Ears!

REVIEW

Discuss what each participant learned, appreciated, and/or applied to their life from last week's session. Any impact on the week's events?

KEY VERSE

"Do not be deceived, my beloved brothers and sisters. Every good thing given and every perfect gift is from above, coming down from the Father of lights, with whom there is no variation or shifting shadow." (James 1:16-17 NASB)

VIDEO STREAMING: SESSION 9

INTRODUCTION

Hopefully, by now, you are beginning to see how confusions, myths, and deceptions about health and wellness can delay our healing, if not downright sabotage it, if we are unaware of the truths. We started by talking about how if a map coordinate was off by just one degree, a plane or a boat could eventually end up way off course. I also addressed how misleading semantics could deter your healing, taking a look at some more common beliefs of "what wellness is not" and "what wellness is." The point was to help you make a paradigm shift in your thinking.

Hopefully, by now, you are also beginning to realize a big difference between the disease management model and the health restoration approach. The disease management model basically alters lab values and helps symptoms go away, primarily utilizing drugs and, at times, medical procedures. The wholistic approach uncovers the root cause of the health imbalance and works towards restoring the body to good health using natural methods.

This session looks at some of the more common differences between the two approaches: the concept of assessing calories versus true nutritional need; allergies versus hidden food sensitivities (semantics again); the truth about real salt; and our body's need for hydrochloric acid, as opposed to suppressing its need. We also highlight the differences between quality supplements and mass-produced synthetic products. The book dives into a few stories and experiences of patients and customers misunderstanding what true health and wellness is all about. These are included to bring continual awareness to how these seemingly minor nuances and misunderstandings can hinder our healing in big ways.

Read Chapter 9 of *Achieving True Wellness in a World of Health Lies* and answer the following questions:

> ➢ If you are currently taking supplements, write an inventory of what you are taking, including the brand and where you bought/buy them.

- Do any of them need to be replaced? Yes/No   _____
- Do any of them need to be eliminated? Yes/No   _____

Put an "X" beside the ones to replace and strike a line through the ones to eliminate.

NOTE: If you got your supplements through a licensed wholistic practitioner, I suggest you keep them. But if you bought them from a friend who told you they are the newest miracle cure, they are most likely a multi-level marketing product. This could mean your friend is making money from selling to you, and someone else is making money from them. I would think twice about these products' "claim to fame." You can most likely find a comparable quality brand that costs less, probably far less, and works just as well. Just because your friend is—well, your friend—doesn't make a supplement a quality product. Ask yourself (and even them), do they truly understand how the body works wholistically or that wellness does NOT happen by simply taking a magic pill?

Start gradually exchanging your unknown, multi-level marketing, internet, drug store, grocery store, and big box discount store brands for quality supplements. This exercise will go a long way toward truly restoring your body to good health, saving you money in the long run—I promise you!

I encourage you to seek out a functional medicine doc who tests for hidden food sensitivity. Until you identify and remove what is causing inflammation in your body, you will be swimming upstream to achieve good health.

If no practitioners in your area do this, I encourage you to eliminate, at least, these top offenders: gluten/wheat, dairy (from cows), sugar, and possibly eggs.

- Do you drink soda? Yes/No   _____
- If so, how much? _____ per day/week/month

If you do nothing else after reading the book, please cut out all sodas from your diet—forever! It just might save your life. I know it might not be easy, so start slowly, and don't stop until you have finally given up ALL sodas. It doesn't matter if it is dark, light, sugar-free (well, it does matter if it's sugar-free, because this is the worst kind of soda!), zero calories—whatever.

> Write out a plan, stick to it, and save your life. This is no exaggeration.

_____
_____
_____

> If you eat margarine, switch to butter—plain and simple.

Have you given authority over your health to God or someone else? If someone else, who?

_____
_____
_____

> Are you happy with your decision? Yes/No?

If not, make a plan to change it. Write down who will have authority over your health.

_____
_____
_____

> Read Robert Young's book, *Sick and Tired, Reclaim Your Inner Terrain*, or his other book, *The pH Miracle*. These can be an additional resource to give you more insight into how you can bring your body BACK to good health—naturally, without drugs or surgeries. When you make these changes, *you* control your health, not the insurance companies, the drug companies, your employer, or the government (Heaven forbid!), etc.

Take an inventory of everything you do that contributes to taking care of your health wholistically. Include chiropractic care; water, including filters for an ionizer, bottled water, other kinds of filters; supplements; massage—anything and everything.

_____

_____

_____

Know how much you are investing in your health. Beside each tool you just listed, write the monthly cost. Guard this part of your budget with all you have. It should take higher priority over cars, homes, clothes, vacations, luxuries, etc. A reasonable budget for a safe place to live and a reliable mode of transportation should be second. Remember, your health is your greatest commodity. Without your health, you won't be able to work to provide for that roof over your head and that car to drive. YOU are highly valuable—irreplaceable, actually.

Are you doing your part toward doing everything possible to take care of your health before looking to other resources to do so? Yes/No _____

- ➤ If you answered "No," write what you can do within your responsibility and control to start taking care of your health.

_____

_____

_____

- ➤ Make a list of what you are not doing but would like to commit to implementing. Write the monthly cost beside each. Write your "start by" date beside each one, in order of priority.

_____

_____

_____

LET'S GO DEEPER

Write any scripture references that God brings to your heart as you ponder the answers to the following questions:

➢ What is God's Word saying to you about being deceived?

_____

_____

_____

➢ Read James 1:12-18. How is the Lord speaking to you about what the world says about sickness and disease versus His truth about wellness through this scripture?

_____

_____

_____

➢ Where are you feeling challenged by or resistant to some of these considerations? What is God speaking to you about that resistance?

_____

_____

_____

➢ What does Isaiah 42:6-7 say to you as it applies to your eyes being opened to the truth?

_____

_____

_____

➢ What is one thing that was an "ah-ha" moment for you that you feel you could grab hold of and own?

➢ What is one change you will commit to moving forward as a result of today's lesson?

➢ What emotions were triggered for you as each of these truths was brought to light?

➢ Why do you think it would be important to God that you commit to making a change in your health based on what you learned from this lesson?

CALL TO ACTION

Consider getting a hidden food sensitivity test. Seek out a functional medicine practitioner to do this for you—conventional medicine is not familiar with it, nor will insurance cover it.

SUMMARY

- Root Cause vs. Disease Management
- Nutrition vs. Calories
- Nutritionist vs. Dietician
- Allergies vs. Hidden Food Sensitivities
- Butter or Margarine?
- Who is the Authority on our Health: God or Modern Medicine?
- Health Comes from Above, Down; Inside, Out
- Are We Enabling Sickness?
- Not Enough Stomach Acid or Too Much?
- The Truth About Salt

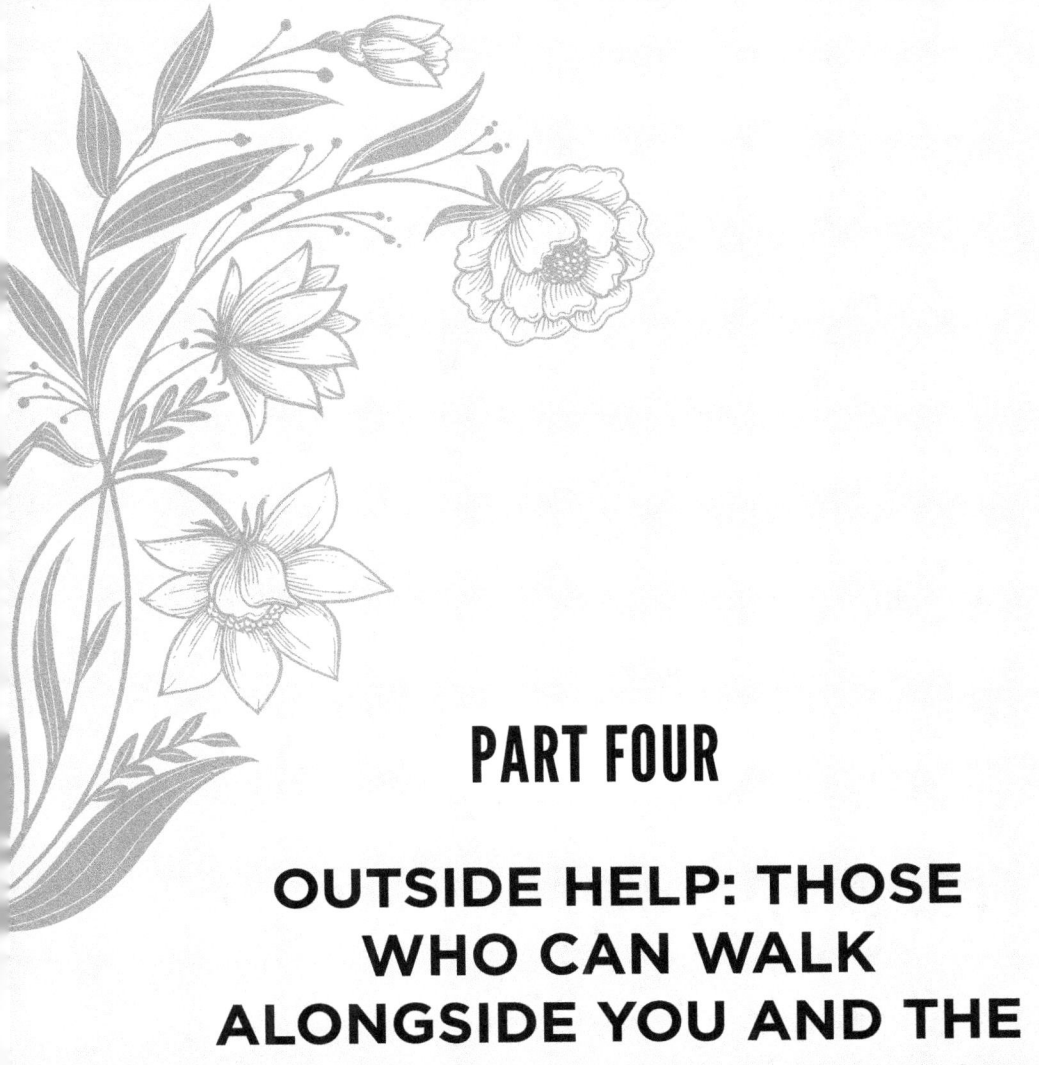

PART FOUR

OUTSIDE HELP: THOSE WHO CAN WALK ALONGSIDE YOU AND THE TOOLS AVAILABLE TO YOU

CHAPTER 10

The Truth About Natural Healthcare Practitioners, Building Your Healthcare Team

REVIEW

Discuss what each participant learned, appreciated, and/or applied to their life from last week's session. Any impact on the week's events?

KEY VERSE

"Just as each one of you has received a special gift [a spiritual talent, an ability graciously given by God], employ it in serving one another as [is appropriate for] good stewards of God's multifaceted grace [faithfully using the diverse, varied gifts and abilities granted to Christians by God's unmerited favor]."
(1 Peter 4:10 AMP)

VIDEO STREAMING: SESSION 10

INTRODUCTION

Establishing your healthcare team in the wholistic world has a different benefit than having an exhausting list of "ologists." In the conventional world, you might have a primary care doctor, a rheumatologist, a gastroenterologist, a cardiologist, a gynecologist, and as you get older, you might even have a gerontologist! The problem here lies in the sad fact that while we *think* they are communicating with each other about our health, they aren't very effective at it. Their primary objective is to address your particular symptom within *their* field of expertise. If another part of the body starts failing, they will refer you to someone else. To sum up: they manage the disease, not the patient. But the wholistic, functional medicine world is the exact opposite. Functional medicine and the wholistic practitioner's primary cohesive objective is to help *you*, the patient, the person as a whole. While conventional medicine practitioners primarily operate in silos, wholistic practitioners work in an overlapping sphere of wellness with the same objective: to utilize their expertise to support the overall plan, and most importantly, *your* goals, to see you and your body functioning at its optimum. They are serving you, as a whole, with their specialized tools, techniques, and expertise.

I encourage you to start building your wholistic healthcare team now. Start with what you already have. Perhaps you have a massage therapist, a chiropractor, or even both. Chapter 10 elaborates on other functional medicine practitioners you might consider as well. Establishing with as many varied practitioners as possible is never too many. This doesn't mean you have to be under the care of all of them at the same time, but you never know when you might need their area of expertise.

Even as I write this, I am considering making an appointment with a wholistic dentist. I had a root canal done in 2019, and it was after that I started having problems with high blood pressure, high platelets, and red blood cells. There is a direct correlation between toxins getting into the bloodstream from invasive dental work and serious health imbalances. In fact, have you ever heard a dentist talk about the importance of regular dental checkups to keep your cardiovascular health in check? Ever wonder why?

Read Chapter 10 of *Achieving True Wellness in a World of Health Lies* and answer the following questions:

Put a check mark by those who are already on your Wellness Team and an "A" for those you want to add:

Chiropractor	☐	Hydrotherapist	☐
Acupuncturist	☐	Massage Therapist	☐
Functional Medicine Doc	☐	Naturopath	☐
Nutritionist	☐	Thermography	☐
Other	☐		

LET'S GO DEEPER

Write any scripture references that God brings to your heart as you ponder the answers to the following questions:

➤ What is God's Word saying to you about being careful who you partner with when it comes to your health?

_____

_____

_____

➤ Read 1 Peter 4:10 in various versions. What is the Lord speaking to you about partnering with those who have been gifted by Him to help others?

_____

_____

_____

➤ What gifting has God blessed you with that might contribute to bringing the truth about wholistic health and wellness to others?

_____

➤ Where are you feeling challenged by or resistant to some of these considerations? What is God speaking to you about that resistance?

➤ What does Isaiah 42:6-7 say to you as it applies to your eyes being opened to the truth of natural healthcare practitioners and providers?

➤ What is one thing that was an "ah-ha" moment for you that you feel you could grab hold of and own?

➤ What is one change you will commit to moving forward as a result of today's lesson?

➤ What emotions were triggered for you as each of these truths was brought to light?

➢ Why do you think it would be important to God that you commit to making a change in your health based on what you learned from this lesson?

CALL TO ACTION

Start building your wholistic wellness team. Make a list of who you might already have on your roster, even if you have only seen them once. If you like and trust them, keep them on your list and build from there.

Even if you don't feel you need their services at the moment, start researching now. If a time comes when you need them urgently, you won't want to be making decisions from a place of panic. You could even go so far as to schedule a consultation appointment just to get established with them. Interview them—perhaps they looked good online, but once you met them in person, they did not resonate with you.

Above all, pray about establishing a relationship with each one. To whom does God want to render care of the body He created?

SUMMARY

- The natural health world tends to draw healers from all kinds of New Age religions. Some of these practitioners believe *they* are the miracle workers, and it is *their* energy doing the healing. Stay as far away from this as possible—I don't care what kind of results they claim to have. Pray about every single practitioner you choose *before* you go to them, whether conventional or wholistic.

- Chiropractors come in various aspects in terms of how we practice and the tools we use.
- Acupuncturists use a technique for balancing the flow of energy that runs along your nervous system through pathways (called meridians) in your body.
- A true nutritionist doesn't count calories. They look at the nutrients that might be depleted in your body and recommend what foods are best for you.
- The naturopathic practice can include some or all of the following diagnostic and therapeutic modalities: clinical and laboratory diagnostic testing, nutritional medicine, botanical medicine, naturopathic physical medicine (including naturopathic manipulative therapy), public health measures, hygiene, counseling, minor surgery, homeopathy, acupuncture, prescription medication, intravenous and injection therapy, and naturopathic obstetrics (natural childbirth).
- Massage therapy is the manipulation of the body's soft tissues, such as muscles, tendons, ligaments, and skin, by using various degrees of pressure and movement. It is typically performed by a licensed professional called a massage therapist, and it's often used as a treatment for various medical conditions.
- A hydrotherapist is trained and licensed. Cleanliness is vital to their profession. The benefit of utilizing the services of a professional hydrotherapist is that their specialized equipment can cleanse the entire length of the colon.
- Thermography is a high-tech health screening tool (a high-definition infrared camera) that creates a digital map of your body and temperature patterns. These patterns may show abnormalities indicative of inflammation (or abnormal heat spots on the body).

CHAPTER 11

The Truth about Supplements

REVIEW

Discuss what each participant learned, appreciated, and/or applied to their life from last week's session. Any impact on the week's events?

KEY VERSE

"So God said, 'Behold, I have given you every plant yielding seed that is on the surface of the entire earth, and every tree which has fruit yielding seed; it shall be food for you.'"
(Genesis 1:29 AMP)

VIDEO STREAMING: SESSION 11

INTRODUCTION

Here is truth number one about supplements: It's not "what do I take?" it's "what do I do?" This just might be the greatest misconception when it comes to what wholistic health and even functional medicine are all about, and the blame starts with wholistic practitioners and providers of supplements. Just like some chiropractors have promoted themselves as the "go-to" for relieving back and neck pain, primarily because that's what insurance covers, so do those who promote natural healing put misplaced emphasis on all the symptoms and health conditions supplements can help overcome.

But the problem doesn't stop there. In fact, it gets worse. When the general population wants to do better for themselves by not taking prescription drugs, or by coming off of their drugs, they often pick up on the misplaced message of "take this latest and greatest natural product for whatever ails you." They start shopping for these products online, at their local big box store, drug store, or grocery store. Multiple mistakes are made.

There are three important messages I hope you take away from this chapter. Actually, we covered the first one in Chapter 2: "Wellness is NOT taking natural supplements for your symptoms." The second lesson is this: Supplements are just that, a "supplement" to bridge the gap between what your diet lacks and what your body still needs in quality nutrients that it should be getting from your food. The third important message is addressed in this session: There is a big difference between quality supplements and synthetically mass-produced ones.

Read Chapter 11 of *Achieving True Wellness in a World of Health Lies* and answer the following questions:

Put a check mark by any of these foundational supplements you already take. If you are taking them, but they are not quality, put a "C" by it to make a note for yourself that you need to "change" brands. If you are not taking a specific supplement, put an "A" by it for "add."

Probiotic ☐

Full spectrum digestive enzyme ☐

Hydrochloric acid (HCl) ☐
(most people need this)

Multi-vitamins and Minerals ☐

Essential Fatty Acids (EFAs), e.g., Omega 3s, fish oil, etc. ☐

Vitamin D ☐

Magnesium ☐
(Ideally a transdermal one. I like the one made by Mg12)

LET'S GO DEEPER

Write any scripture references that God brings to your heart as you ponder the answers to the following questions:

➤ Read Genesis 1:29 in different versions. What does this verse say to you about the natural healing properties God has blessed us with?

_____

_____

➤ Where are you feeling challenged by or resistant to some of these considerations? What is God speaking to you about that resistance?

_____

_____

➤ What does Isaiah 42:6-7 say to you as it applies to your eyes being opened to the truth about the bounty from the earth that He has blessed us with?

_____

_____

_____

_____

➢ What is one thing that was an "ah-ha" moment for you that you feel you could grab hold of and own?

_____

_____

_____

➢ What is one change you will commit to making moving forward as a result of today's lesson?

_____

_____

_____

➢ What emotions were triggered for you as each of these truths was brought to light?

_____

_____

_____

➢ Why do you think it would be important to God that you commit to making a change in your health based on what you learned from this lesson?

_____

_____

_____

CALL TO ACTION

I encourage you to learn more about those natural products that are unfamiliar to you, like herbal medicine, homeopathy, and mushrooms. If you are not confident in what they can do or how they work, you will probably tend to avoid them. Most likely, they sound a little foreign to you (especially the last two), but they have tremendous healing abilities.

By understanding how they work and what they can do, you can expand the "tools in your wellness toolbox" and utilize them with confidence when you need to.

SUMMARY

- Supplements collectively cover a broad spectrum of subcategories.
- There are two basic categories of vitamins: fat-soluble and water-soluble.
- Vitamins A, D, E, and K are fat-soluble vitamins that dissolve in fat and are stored in the liver and fat tissues until needed.
- Vitamin B-complex and vitamin C are water-soluble vitamins that are dissolved in water and eliminated in urine.
- Magnesium is known as the "master mineral." All other vitamins and minerals need a sufficient quantity and the right form of magnesium to function as God intended.
- The strength and potency of herbs are incredible and many times equal to or even far greater than a drug.
- Homeopathy works on a molecular level along the energetic pathways that make up the nervous system.
- Medicinal mushrooms like Reishi, Maitake, Chaga, Lion's Mane, Cordyceps, and so many more have tremendous healing properties, especially for the immune system, and can even address conditions like cancer.

CHAPTER 12

The Truth about Wholistic Health Tests

REVIEW

Discuss what each participant learned, appreciated, and/or applied to their life from last week's session. Any impact on the week's events?

KEY VERSE

"But test all things carefully [so you can recognize what is good]. Hold firmly to that which is good."
(1 Thessalonians 5:21 AMP)

VIDEO STREAMING: SESSION 12

INTRODUCTION

Everything is relative. Take statistics, for example. I could run a set of numbers and work them to my favor if I really wanted. When I first started selling real estate (yes, I'm a jack of all trades, but master of only a few!), I remember my broker telling me to go out and promote myself as "the #1 agent." Hmmm, but I was not number one, far from it, in fact, and I expressed my concern about "false advertising." His reply was, "Does anyone else in your family sell real estate? Then you ARE the number one agent!" Okay then. It's all relative.

Functional medicine test interpretations versus conventional medicine interpretations are a somewhat similar example of relativity. Not that either one is skewing the actual results. They just view test results from different perspectives. The conventional medicine world looks at labs and other test results to see if there is a disease. The functional medicine world looks at the results to assess the patient as a whole, not as a disease. We also look much more comprehensively at lab values for different objectives.

Cholesterol levels are a classic example. In addition to assessing the state of one's cardiovascular health, in the functional medicine world, we are also looking at the state of the person's liver (where the majority of cholesterol is made) as well as inflammation that might be anywhere in the body, not just the vasculature. Cholesterol is not the bad guy. It simply shows up at the sight of inflammation, so we use this as one of the markers to give us a general inflammatory state of the person, too. Functional medicine is also concerned with cholesterol being too low, i.e., below 140 is an ominous sign to us. Not good! However, I've seen conventional medicine lab values for cholesterol range from 0-200. In other words, a value like 140 would never be on their radar! I know people whose conventional doctors want their cholesterol down to 100 before they will take them off their medication—scary. We need cholesterol. All of our hormones are made up of cholesterol. Our immune system, in part, is made up of cholesterol. And these are just *some* of the many beneficial functions of cholesterol.

This chapter looks at some of the more common differences between conventional medicine and functional medicine when it comes to lab testing.

Read Chapter 12 of *Achieving True Wellness in a World of Health Lies* and answer the following questions:

Look at the latest cholesterol numbers you have. If it has been over a year, I encourage you to go see your primary care doc. Better yet, this could be a good reason to establish care with a wholistic practitioner and ask them to run your cholesterol for you. While you are at it, ask them to run a comprehensive lab panel to establish all your numbers. Keep in mind that, most likely, only a wholistic practitioner will do this for you. Conventional medicine docs only order what the insurance companies allow them to order, i.e., the very basics.

Once you have your cholesterol values in front of you, do the simple math to determine what your coronary risk factor (CRF) is: Total Cholesterol divided by HDL. You want to see 3.0 or less.

Write your CRF here _____

Next, make sure your total cholesterol is over 140. Ideally, over 160. If it's less than 140, I highly encourage you to schedule an appointment with a functional medicine practitioner and express concerns about your cholesterol being too low. Note: a conventional medicine practitioner may very likely not find 140 to be too low, as the current reference range for "healthy" cholesterol has recently been changed to 100-200.

Are you on cholesterol meds? If so, based on what you have learned, do you really need to be? Talk this over with the practitioner who prescribed them. If your lab values are good based on this comprehensive assessment, and they still don't want to take you off these drugs, I encourage you to seek out a second opinion from a functional medicine practitioner.

Remember the risk factors of being on cholesterol meds: they are very toxic to the liver, and they rob the body of the vital antioxidant CoQ10.

Look for a natural healthcare practitioner who will run a 24-hour urine iodine test for you if you suspect you have thyroid problems or have been told you need to go on meds. I hope this chapter has opened your eyes to the truth about thyroid testing.

If you are on medication(s) for depression, anxiety, or other mental health challenges, I can't encourage you enough to please seek out a functional medicine practitioner to run a neurotransmitter test. Anyone I've ever talked with who is on prescription meds prescribed by a traditional practitioner has never had a neurotransmitter test run. They have only ever been managed by subjective input, based on how they felt at any given time, with their meds adjusted accordingly.

LET'S GO DEEPER

- Read 1 Thessalonians 5:21. Where might you be feeling challenged by or resistant to testing what is good?

- What is one thing that was an "ah-ha" moment for you that you feel you could grab hold of and own?

- What is one change you will commit to making moving forward as a result of today's lesson?

- What emotions were triggered for you as each of these truths was brought to light?

➤ Why do you think it would be important to God that you commit to making a change in your health based on what you learned from this lesson?

CALL TO ACTION

If you are on cholesterol meds based on your total cholesterol and/or your LDL being high, or if your CRF number is greater than 3.0, I suggest having a VAP test run to learn what the particle sizes of the cholesterol are. It is quite common that some who have what looks like a "normal" cholesterol reading have a positive VAP test, while others who have what looks like high cholesterol have a negative (or good) VAP test.

If you are on thyroid meds based on the basic thyroid labs, go back to the prescribing doctor and insist on a complete and comprehensive thyroid panel that includes (but is not limited to) the thyroid antibodies TPO and TGB. If they will not do this for you, find another practitioner—ideally, a functional medicine doc who will assess your thyroid completely and accurately.

If you are on antidepressants and/or anxiety meds, I highly encourage you to seek out a functional medicine doctor who will order a neurotransmitter test for you.

SUMMARY

- The most important number on the cholesterol panel should be the CRF or Total-to-HDL ratio.

- Our bodies need cholesterol since all of our hormones are made up of cholesterol. To operate properly, our bodies must have our hormones functioning properly.

- Cholesterol is not usually the root cause of clogged arteries—it's inflammation.

- A better test to determine your coronary risk, where cholesterol is concerned, is called a VAP test.

- Every cell in the body needs iodine. The thyroid, breast tissue, uterus, ovaries, and testicles all need a heavy saturation of iodine. However, most people are actually deficient in it.

- A Comprehensive Digestive Stool Analysis (CDSA) test checks the levels of good and bad bacteria, good and bad levels of yeast, the presence of parasites (more Americans have parasites than realize it!), gut intolerances to certain foods, the absorption capabilities of the gut, and so much more.

- Neurotransmitters are our brain hormones or brain chemicals. These include epinephrine, norepinephrine, dopamine, serotonin, GABA, and acetylcholine in particular, as well as hormones like leptin and ghrelin (the brain chemicals that regulate our appetite) and melatonin.

- A neurotransmitter test can first tell us at the levels of each of these neurotransmitters and hormones. From there, we can assess which ones are too high, which are too low, and address them accordingly.

Conclusion

I now invite you to take the health and wellness knowledge you came into this course with back off the shelf and see how it compares to these new insights you've learned over the past 12 sessions.

Give thought once again to which path you will pursue: Disease management or health restoration? What is *your* objective for your health? If it is to pursue health restoration, then congratulations, you have chosen LIFE!

I would like to leave you with these words of encouragement: your health IS in your control. It's empowering, and it's FREEDOM!

My prayer for you is that you continue applying what you have learned from this book, the workbook, and the video course. It's a process. In fact, it's a life-changing process. If you fall off the horse, simply get back on. None of us is perfect, and we WILL fall off from time to time. Proverbs 24:16 says, *"The godly may trip seven times, but they will get up again. But one disaster is enough to overthrow the wicked."* Through God's grace and mercy, when we depend on Him for all things, including our health, we *can* and *will* overcome the darts of the enemy, which are sickness and disease. A righteous man or woman gets back up and overcomes.

APPENDIX A

Suggested Reading and Resources

Books

What to Say When You Talk to Yourself – Shad Helmstetter, PhD

True Confessions of an Rx Drug Pusher – Gwen Olsen

Death by Medicine – Gary Null, Ph.D

Food & Behavior, A Natural Connection – Barbara Reed Stitt

Why is My Brain Not Working? – Datis Kharrazian, DHSc., DC, MS

No More Dirty Looks – Siobhan O'Connor & Alexandra Spunt

How to Hear God's Voice – Mark Virkler

Sick & Tired? Reclaim Your Inner Terrain – Dr. Robert Young

The pH Miracle, Balance Your Diet, Reclaim Your Health – Dr. Robert Young

Hope Medicine & Healing – Francisco Contreras, MD & Daniel E. Kennedy, MC

Beyond Gluten Intolerance – Karen Masterson Koch, CN

The Miracle of Magnesium – Dr. Carolyn Dean

The Healing Revolution – Dr. Frank King

Why Stomach Acid is Good for You – Jonathan V. Wright, M.D. & Lane Lenard, Ph.D.

Salt Your Way to Health – David Brownstein, M.D.

Overcoming Thyroid Disorders – David Brownstein, M.D.

MycoMedicinals: An Informational Treatise on Mushrooms – Paul Stamets

Your Body's Many Cries for Water – F. Batmanghelidj, M.D.

Gut Solutions – Brenda Watson, N.D.

Back to Eden – Jethro Kloss

Salt, Sugar, Fat – Michael Moss

Raw Food & Alkalizing Recipe Books

Raw Food, A Complete Guide for Every Meal of the Day – Erica Palmcrantz and Irmelda Lilja

The Hallelujah Diet: Experience the Optimal Health You Were Meant to Have – George Malkmus

Everyday Raw – Matthew Kenney

Ani's Raw Food Essentials – Ani Phyo

Alkaline Diet Recipe Book (Volumes I & II) – Ross Bridgeford

Businesses/Organizations

Mg12 Magnesium – www.mg12.com – use code TAW for a 10% discount

Oasis of Hope Cancer Treatment Center – https://www.oasisofhope.com/

Gaia Herbs Farm – https://www.gaiaherbs.com/pages/our-farm

Frontier Co-op – https://www.frontiercoop.com/

Alliance for Natural Health – https://anh-usa.org/

Communion With God Ministries, at www.cwgministries.org

Dave Ramsey, Financial Peace University – www.ramseysolutions.com

Cleansing Stream – www.cleansingstream.org

Healing Rooms Ministries – www.healingrooms.com

Hallelujah Acres – https://myhdiet.com/blogs/healthnews

Resources for Finding Wholistic Practitioners

The American Chiropractic Association's Council on Diagnosis and Internal Disorders (CDID)
https://www.acacdid.com/searchdoctors

The Chiropractic Board of Clinical Nutrition
https://www.cbcn.us/diplomate-directory

The American Clinical Board of Nutrition (ACBN)
https://www.acbn.org/

American Nutrition Association
https://theana.org/

The Institute for Functional Medicine
https://www.ifm.org/find-a-practitioner/

Functional Medicine University
https://www.functionalmedicineuniversity.com/public/find-Functional-Medicine-Clinicians.cfm

APPENDIX B

WHOLISTIC GOALS

MENTAL

Goal:

Action Steps:

EMOTIONAL

Goal:

Action Steps:

PHYSICAL

Goal:

Action Steps:

SPIRITUAL

Goal:

Action Steps:

APPENDIX C

FOOD LOG

The purpose of this Food Log is not only to keep track of all the foods you eat on a daily and weekly basis, but also to bring awareness to what and how often you are (or are not) eating. Remember my Cheez-its story?

List in detail the quantity and the exact nature of all foods and beverages consumed (i.e., frozen, canned, etc.). Please mention if the foods were raw or cooked. Be sure to list any condiments (e.g., mayonnaise, margarine, relish, etc.).

MEAL	DAY 1	DATE

Morning Meal:

Time:

Snack:

Noon Meal:

Time:

Snack:

Evening Meal:

Time:

Snack: _____

Water (ounces per day)_____

Other Beverages (type and amount):_____

MEAL	DAY 2	DATE

Morning Meal:

Time:

Snack: _____

Noon Meal:

Time:

Snack: _____

Evening Meal:

Time:

Snack: _____

Water (ounces per day) _____

Other Beverages (type and amount): _____

MEAL	DAY	DATE

Morning Meal:

Time:

Snack: _____

Noon Meal:

Time:

Snack: _____

Evening Meal:

Time:

Snack: _____

Water (ounces per day)_____

Other Beverages (type and amount): _____

MEAL	DAY 4	DATE

Morning Meal:

Time:

Snack: _____

Noon Meal:

Time:

Snack: _____

Evening Meal:

Time:

Snack: _____

Water (ounces per day)_____

Other Beverages (type and amount): _____

MEAL	DAY 5	DATE

Morning Meal:

Time:

_____
 Snack:
_____

Noon Meal:

Time:

_____
 Snack:
_____

Evening Meal:

Time:

_____
 Snack:
_____

Water (ounces per day)_____

Other Beverages (type and amount): _____

| MEAL | DAY 6 | DATE |

Morning Meal:

Time:

Snack: _____

Noon Meal:

Time:

Snack: _____

Evening Meal:

Time:

Snack: _____

Water (ounces per day)_____

Other Beverages (type and amount): _____

| MEAL | DAY 4 | DATE |

Morning Meal:

Time:

Snack:

Noon Meal:

Time:

Snack:

Evening Meal:

Time:

Snack:

Water (ounces per day)_____

Other Beverages (type and amount): _____

About Dr. Jackie McKool

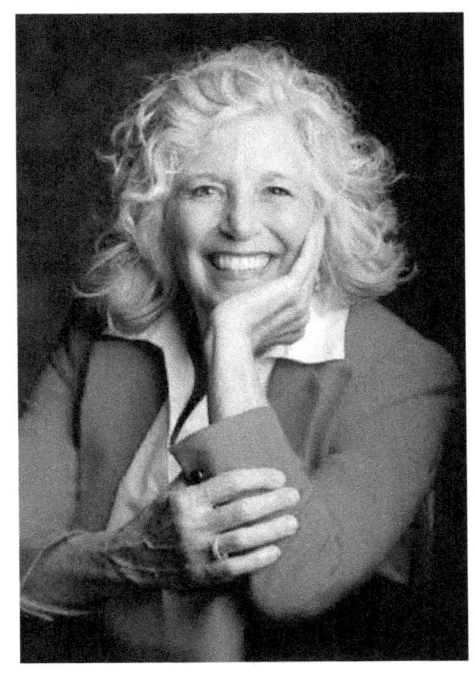

Dr. Jackie McKool has been passionate about wholistic health and wellness since God delivered her in 1996 from an addiction to alcohol. He pulled her out of the miry clay and set her feet on a new path—a wholistic path of health and healing. She believes with all her heart and soul that God has called her to speak, teach, and write with the purpose of glorifying Him.

Dr. McKool spent 10 years in the wholistic health and wellness field as a chiropractic physician in Charleston, South Carolina. She has her post-doctorate in Internal Disorders, making her one of fewer than 500 worldwide board-certified Chiropractic Internists with a focus on Internal Disorders. Upon moving to North Carolina, she worked in the natural products industry in several health food stores.

Dr. McKool has served as a trained minister for several Christian healing ministries, including Cleansing Stream, founded by Pastor Jack Hayford, and the International Healing Rooms Ministries, founded by Reverend Cal Pierce. She has also studied under Dr. Mark Virkler, founder of Christian Leadership University and Communion with God Ministries. Dr. Virkler is also the author of *4 Keys to Hearing God's Voice*.

In addition to wholistic health and wellness, Dr. McKool loves being in God's creation outdoors. She claims she was "born to be outside!" She loves jogging, hiking, biking, kayaking, and most of all, backpacking. At the age of 65, she completed her 11-year journey of backpacking the Appalachian Trail (AT), a 2,200-mile-long foot trail, by summiting Mt. Katahdin on August 11th, 2024. Look for her next book, that is already brewing about her adventures on the AT!

She lives in western North Carolina with her two fur baby cats, KoKo and Sadie.

To reach Dr. Jackie for speaking opportunities or to follow her blog:

www.jackiemckool.com
jackie@jackiemckool.com
www.facebook.com/drjackiemckool

www.ingramcontent.com/pod-product-compliance
Lightning Source LLC
Chambersburg PA
CBHW081454070526
44586CB00019B/2346